Speech Teacher:

A Random Narrative

Loren Reid

Published by the
Speech Communication Association
Annandale, Virginia
1990

Library of Congress Catalog Card Number: 90-063139
ISBN: 0-944811-05-1

First published in November 1990

Speech Communication Association, 5105 Backlick Road, Building E, Annandale, VA 22003

Printed in the United States of America.

Contents

Foreword

The Speech Communication Association (SCA) is proud to be able to publish *Speech Teacher: A Random Narrative*. This publication contributes the experiences of Loren Reid, a former Executive Secretary and President of SCA, to a growing list of historically-oriented publications that began in 1943 with the publication of the two volume *A History of American Public Address*, edited by William Norwood Brigance.

Previous histories of SCA

SCA continued to publish historical volumes in the 1950's. For example, under the editorship of Karl R. Wallace, *History of Speech Education in America* was published in 1954. Under the editorship of Marie Kathryn Hochmuth [Nichols], the third volume of *A History and Criticism of American Public Address* was published in 1955.

SCA's 50th anniversary in 1964 renewed the Association's interest in its history. The *Quarterly Journal of Speech* devoted pages to this landmark in the history of the Association. "The Founding of the Speech Association of America: Happy Birthday" by Giles W. Gray describes the historical moments which gave birth to the Speech Communication Association. "A History of the Speech Association of America, 1914-1964" by Robert C. Jeffrey reviewed specific patterns of growth and development in the Association.

The Association also published *Speech Association of America Golden Anniversary 1964* which included contemporary articles and several reprints from the *Quarterly Journal of Speech* which captured the history of the Association.

With the observance of the 75th anniversary of the Association last year came several new publications. The Association sponsored an edited volume by Gerald M. Phillips and Julia A. Wood entitled *Speech Communication: Essays to Commemorate the 75th Anniversary of the Speech Communication Association*. This publication provides a series of state-of-the-art reviews of major content areas defining the discipline of speech communication.

A second publication in 1989 entitled *The Past Is Prologue: A 75th Anniversary Publication of the Speech Communication Association* focused on the history of the Association. Edited by William Work and Robert C. Jeffrey, the volume contains reprints of earlier historical essays as well as new and updated articles tracing the growth of the Association and the discipline.

SCA's 75th anniversary was also celebrated with a special retrospective issue of *Time* magazine, titled *Communication 1940-1989*. The magazine includes news accounts and photographs of significant events in the history of communication. The articles and photos were selected from the *Time* magazine archives and related to the history of the discipline by J. Jeffery Auer, Robert C. Jeffrey, Gerald R. Miller, Patti P. Gillespie, and Carolyn Calloway-Thomas.

SCA's 75th anniversary also motivated the publication of Theodore Otto Windt, Jr.'s *Rhetoric as a Human Adventure: A Short Biography of Everett Lee Hunt*. *Rhetoric as a Human Adventure* traces the intellectual and professional growth of Hunt, a man who began as a teacher of oratory and a coach of debate at a small sectarian college in North Dakota, matured at the Cornell School of Rhetoric and ended his career as Dean of Swarthmore. Windt writes of a friend and a scholar who actively participated in the early debates that helped to shape our discipline and our Association.

Speech Teacher

In *Speech Teacher: A Random Narrative* Loren Reid writes of his experiences as a speech teacher, first at Vermillion (SD) High School and later at the University of Missouri and Syracuse University. Along the way, he provides interesting and often humorous accounts of such events as his first SCA convention (in Chicago), his Ph.D. studies and dissertation, his first convention paper, and his life as a speech teacher during the WWII era.

Speech Teacher is, however, more than an autobiographical account of his professional life; it is also a history of the discipline and of SCA. Chapter titles such as "Elocution, Speech and Shakespeare" and "If You Love 'Em, Join 'Em" describe his and the profession's transition from English to Speech.

In the chapter titled "The Original Gold Card Era" he describes the problems he faced as the SCA Executive Secretary during the post war era, such as finding hotel space for conventions and purchasing paper to print the Association's publications.

Loren Reid was not at the convention of the National Association of Teachers of English during which 17 members — the "Founding Fathers" — broke away to form the National Association of Academic Teachers of Public Speaking, later to become SCA. He was of the second generation of leaders that followed, and he played an important role in shaping the discipline and the Association. *Speech Teacher* is the story of his contribution to the generations that will follow him.

James L. Gaudino
Executive Director
Speech Communication Association
September 1990

Preface

The writing of this book was motivated by the Diamond Anniversary of the Speech Communication Association in 1989. To exist seventy-five years, and especially to enjoy steady growth, is no mean achievement.

During the twentieth century the art and science of communication expanded and changed in ways that we could not have dreamed of. For no good reason, except that it is the year of my birth, I start with 1905. Theodore Roosevelt, the youngest ever President, communicated well enough to win a gubernatorial and two presidential elections, and along the way to become a Nobel peace prize winner. Another outstanding speaker was William Jennings Bryan; though he lost three presidential elections, he continued as a dominant figure in his party. He talked to tens of thousands of people, a few hundred or more at a time, just as Abe Lincoln and Judge Douglas and Frederick Douglass and Susan B. Anthony had.

In 1914, the National Association of Academic Teachers of Public Speaking was founded in Chicago by 17 men, to be known as the Founding Fathers. By then the telegraph was not only transcontinental but transatlantic, and the telephone became transcontinental a short time after the new Association was founded. I was in fifth grade, living in Gilman City, a northwest Missouri community of 600. Late afternoons and sometimes evenings I worked in the family newspaper, the *Gilman City Guide*. I did not realize when I was running a Linotype and printing sale bills and writing news stories that I was training to become a professor of speech. The speakers who came to enlighten the community—a candidate for the State House, or Congress, or the Senate—did not know about electric amplifiers but they did know that they should call on Father, the *Guide* editor, to get a free write-up. At school I participated in the speaking activities the school offered—a Friday afternoon program, a Christmas skit, a debate on a local issue such as whether raising mules was more profitable than raising hogs.

When Woodrow Wilson made his critical campaign for reelection in 1916 (the new Association then being two years old) the whole town gathered at the depot to listen to the reports that telegraph operators around the country poured into the general network. Anything else we needed to know we could learn from the *Kansas City Star* or the *St. Joseph News-Press* which arrived every day on the noon train. When as President he took his plea for a League of Nations to the people, he traveled by train from one city to another, talking to immense crowds without benefit of public address systems. Some of what he said would be relayed through the news reels at the theaters. We had little trouble in keeping well-informed.

I will not repeat here the story of how those 17 men met in a Chicago hotel and organized the National Association of Academic Teachers of Public Speaking. "Academic" set them apart from "elocutionists" who worked through private studios. I call the Founders and their contemporaries the first generation of academic teachers of communication. Calling them the "first" is capricious, as there has been a long history of people who taught some kind of speech in some kind of school, but it is a way of organizing what has happened since 1905, give or take a few years. Very few of the Founding Fathers and their contemporaries had a Ph.D. in any field, much less in any form of communication. Their students, whose careers started in the 1930s, became the second generation; most of them had retired by the time of the Diamond Anniversary convention; and the young men and women who are now in the saddle, at the steering wheel, on the mountain top looking through the telescope, are the third generation. More of this later.

The first Ph.D. in this new field was awarded in 1922. It was a day in 1922 that a high school senior was walking across the courthouse park in his new home of Osceola, Iowa. He stopped to join three boys who were tinkering with the cat's hair of a crystal radio, and finally heard a crackling sound of distant music. The first licensed radio broadcast had been in 1920, so it had taken a while for radio sets to get to Osceola. Radio, and later television, expanded the ways in which people could communicate, thus opening up whole new fields of expertise. And of teaching. Before mid-century a New Yorker by the name of Franklin Delano Roosevelt had shown the country how to use radio to unite and to lead a nation through a dreary depression and a world war. If you want other names, how about Eleanor Roosevelt, Winston Churchill, Charles de Gaulle, John F. Kennedy, Martin Luther King. The rapid developments in television are known to all; we have talked to the moon and back; we get pictures of distant planets; and as we end the century we can note that thousands of fifth graders know that word processors can be linked into networks that go everywhere.

Most of what I write is about this second generation of teachers, who, given these amazing new tools of communication, built their own networks of regional and state associations. They persuaded high schools, colleges, and universities to create new departments to study and practice the principles of communication. They led the fight to get approval for master's and doctor's degrees and thus brought the field into the academic world.

More Preface

In writing this narrative, I have had in the back of my mind the thought that most people are in one way inside persons and in another way outside persons.

As inside persons, teachers are involved with classes and students, lesson plans, experiments, ways of presenting information and concepts, and, at times, wisdom. We are counselors, advisers, sponsors. We introduce students to prospective employers. Sometimes we advise on personal matters. We are mentors— after Mentor, the friend to whom Odysseus entrusted the education of his son. As teachers we are ourselves students, in the basic sense of the word—*student* carries the root meaning of *eager, enthusiastic*. Some of this root meaning carries over into an expression such as "She is a real student of baseball," meaning that she is an avid lover of the game and knows its history and its people. This enthusiasm leads us to learn more about a topic than we will ever teach in a class.

Any given teacher may participate in church or community activities, in conventions and conferences of state, regional, and national associations, and in so doing becomes an outside person. It is the old rule of sailing ships—"one hand for yourself, one hand for the ship." One hand to hold on, so when the big blows come you will not be washed into the sea—if that happens, you are lost, and the ship has lost your services. One hand for the ship—the lines, the sails, the rudder, must be kept operating lest the ship founder and everything disappear.

Either career is fully rewarding. As the years go on, teachers-as-students realize that their influence was more profound than they realized. Teachers outside the classroom find that sometimes they get more credit for an outside interest than for their inside interest. What I have written applies to all walks of life. Here is an actor who races automobiles and also has a profound interest in charities. Here is an Olympic champion who works with underprivileged boys and girls in her home town. At a social group your known expertise is taken for granted; what amazes your listeners is the sudden discovery that you are a Civil War buff and that you "collect" Civil War battlefields.

This narrative is about classes, which is an inside story, and about organizations, which is an outside story. I write as a member of the generation of teachers of speech that happened to be around when the discipline was rapidly reaching out.

Loren Reid
Columbia, Missouri
1990

1

In the Beginning

I begin this narrative, which is indeed random, by noting that others could have told it better, but many of them are not here; that many who are here will freely supplement it; and that those who follow will read what we eventually get written. Many of those who follow will modestly reflect, What a lot happened even before we got here.

I begin as another Missourian once did: "You don't know about me, without you have read a book by the name of *The Adventures of Tom Sawyer*, but that ain't no matter. That book was made by Mr. Mark Twain, and he told the truth mainly. There was things which he stretched, but mainly he told the truth." You don't know about me, without you have a read a book by the name of *Hurry Home Wednesday: Growing Up in a Small Missouri Town, 1905-1920*. I tell about early days as member of a newspaper family in Gilman City, population 619, northwest Missouri, doing everything from reporting to Linotyping. I also mention debating and oratorical contests. There was things which I stretched, but mainly I told the truth. Much of what I was to do later was based on this experience with a mass medium called *The Gilman City Guide*, circulation 452.

I showed the manuscript of *Hurry Home Wednesday* to the University of Missouri Press, which did not want to publish a title without any footnotes whatever, but the staff finally took a deep breath and brought it out, late at night, under the cover of darkness. I wrote a sequel, *Finally It's Friday: School and Work in Mid-America, 1921-1933*, telling how I left newspaperdom and entered teaching, deciding at first to teach English, but then speech. Generally, but not always, I use the term "speech" to include theater and speech pathology as well as public speaking and rhetoric (in the early years all of us taught in the same department, drank coffee at the same snack bar, and attended the same conventions). Any graduate student of the current day who thinks doctoral study in our discipline is tough (which it is) may thankfully reflect that he or she avoided graduate study in the 1930s, which was not only tough but at times seemed impossible.

I HAVE ALWAYS regretted that I did not attend that famous convention of the National Association of Teachers of English in Chicago, at which 17 men broke away to organize the National Association of Academic Teachers of Public Speaking—NAATPS for short—which, after two name changes, became the Speech Communication Association. It would be nice, now that I can look back on 75 years of activity, and forward to 100 and more, to be viewed with amazement as one of the founders.

As already mentioned, I was then living in Gilman City, and could easily have made the trip to Chicago. The cost would have been modest; at the going rate of a cent a mile, $6.00 would have covered the train fare. A room at the convention hotel, The Auditorium, was $1.50, if I were willing to accept a "detached bath," which I always was. I could have eaten splendidly for $1.50 a day. So much for the logistics.

In part my failure to be present was because the meeting was really not well advertised. A mere 60 had made it to the preliminary discussion, and of those, only 17 showed up for the adjourned session at which the critical, historic decision was taken. And besides, I was only in fifth grade.

Of the 17, among those who became especially well known to the profession were: Frank M. Rarig, University of Minnesota, age 34; Lew Sarett, Northwestern University, 26; James M. O'Neill, University of Wisconsin, 33; Charles H. Woolbert, University of Illinois, 37; James M. Winans, Cornell University,

43. I have called these men and the rest of the 17, and contemporaries like my doctoral adviser A. Craig Baird of the University of Iowa, Lena E. Misener of the El Reno, Okla., High School, Andrew T. Weaver of the University of Wisconsin, Ralph B. Dennis of Northwestern University, Maud May Babcock of the University of Utah, Henrietta Prentiss of Hunter College, and a hundred or so others, not forgetting my high school debate coach, Lois Graham, the first generation of academically-based speech teachers, the generation that followed the teachers of elocution. As for the founding fathers, my generation, as young men and women, were to know all but two or three of them. We could speak of "Jim" O'Neill or "Chief" Winans or "Charley" Woolbert.

If you do not recognize any of these names, don't let it worry you. If you were conversing with a group of your contemporaries, and the talk went gently back to the earlier years of your home town, or business, or profession, or some sport, like baseball, you would produce your own cluster of names—some of them heroic, some of them not.

The new NAATPS held its first convention in Chicago in 1915, with 60 members present. The second meeting at The Astor, in New York, attracted 80. For the third meeting it returned to Chicago in The Congress ($2.00 and up). Treasurer H. S. Woodward reported that more than 100 were there, although only 84 actually registered—an early instance of attending a convention but skipping the fee ($1.00). Those 84 represented 15 states, 78 institutions.[1] Half of them came from distances no farther than Gilman City was.

By 1920, the NAATPS had increased its membership from 160 to 700. Gilman City increased its population more slowly, holding at 619; I had made it all the way from fifth grade to high school sophomore. That year my favorite teacher was Lois Graham, beautiful and charming daughter of a physician in nearby Jamesport; she taught English and Latin. In addition to the usual teaching credentials of a couple of years at one of the State Normal Colleges, Miss Lois had studied elocution at the Cumnock School, which became the School of Speech at Northwestern University. Many midwestern teachers had studied elocution at the Emerson School or the Curry School in Boston, but we were led to believe that Cumnock was superior, and we faithfully followed the exercises Miss Lois gave us, generally aimed at getting us to soften our midwestern r's and to pronounce *aunt* more like "ahnt" than *ant*.

Because of this remote connection, I should say a word about Robert McLean Cumnock. He came to Northwestern in 1868, taught until 1913, then retired from active teaching. In 45 years he never missed a class. Surely this statement is a stretcher, but I did not originate it. In 1878 he organized a School of Oratory as part of Northwestern. For a while this was called a School of Oratory and Physical Education. Cumnock was called "a heroic figure from an earlier age." Fastidious in his dress, he hated slovenly speech. His singleness of purpose was "to teach men and women to speak accurately and nobly." "Nobly" is a word we hardly use any more. He died in 1928, at the age of 88.[2] I could have met him, but never did; in the 1940s, however, I taught in a university where the two oldest professors still proudly used his book, *Choice Readings*; they had seen no reason to switch.

In *Hurry Home Wednesday*, I describe taking part in the annual oratorical contest:

> Miss Lois spent hours after school coaching the contestants. My practice period came between that of a girl who was reciting a sad story about Bobby Shaftoe, who had gone to sea, but who will come back and marry me, and that of a boy with a robust voice, whose selection by Webster about John Adams ended with the thunderous note, "It [the Declaration] is my living sentiment, and by the blessing of God, it shall be my dying sentiment; independence now and independence forever." I secretly had him tagged as the winner, since by contrast the quiet poetry of Col. Bob Ingersoll, my piece, seemed a frail thing.[3]

The night of the contest, however, Col. Bob prevailed over the godlike Daniel, and I advanced to the district contest. In further preparation, Father took me for an extra lesson with a teacher at Trenton, a half-hour train ride to the east. This teacher, also in the Cumnock tradition, wisely did not make drastic changes but, interestingly enough, would stop me now and then to ask me "what I meant by" phrases like "sunshine patriot"; and if a sunshine patriot were really one who fought only when the cause was winning and not when the going was tough, could I suggest all that by the way I spoke. On the way home Father and I discussed her suggestions and decided the time and money had been well invested. I am not sure about Cumnock's "noble" part but am fairly certain about the "accurate" part.

I won the district, but only second in the regional, which rained on my parade to the state championship. Though I was disappointed, I decided to try out for debate, the question at the time being whether compulsory arbitration between employer and employee was wise and feasible. As our first opponent we drew Martinsville, a tiny town in the west part of the county. The Gilman City superintendent and the Martinsville superintendent sparred over the selection of judges, but finally, by offering to host the debate and lodge the visitors, our superintendent got what he considered was an edge in selecting the three judges. The following is lifted from *Hurry Home Wednesday*:

A few days before the debate, I had read an account of an experiment involving a man whose stomach had been opened by a gunshot wound. Every viewer of westerns knows that to be gut-shot is to invite a sure and painful death, but this victim escaped that ordeal and endured another. For a reason not clear, the attending surgeon, instead of promptly sewing him up, left the hole open in his stomach to observe the digestive process. The surgeon fed his interesting patient, for example, oatmeal, and then recorded the length of time the oatmeal was in the stomach. Roast beef, I recall, lay three hours and forty minutes in the stomach before being emptied into the small intestine. Roast pork was the most difficult of all; four hours and forty minutes. Other items were also listed.

I rushed the book into the superintendent's office. Like any German, he loved good food, and his wife was a superb cook. He immediately grasped the significance of what I showed him. Since as hosts we were obliged to provide the Martinsville debaters with supper, we would select a meal from the table of digestive times. Everybody knew that blood was siphoned from the brain after a heavy meal. Very well, we would stuff the visitors with proper foods, leading with roast pork.

The great day arrived. At the supper table were the four debaters and their coaches. Two of our most bewitching classmates, fully briefed on the plan, waited on the table. They made sure that our guests had plenty of the main course and the supplements, including fried, browned potatoes and thick, rich gravy, all German style. Manipulation may be new in our consciousness today, but the practice is reasonably ancient. We ate sparingly. The visitors rose from the table goggle-eyed. The party had to hurry to get to the Rex Theater on time.

The theater was packed. . . . Each debater was applauded. When the debate was over, the audience buzzed excitedly. A contest could hardly be closer; the decision could truly go either way. . . . On our side . . . we had countered every argument with something, we had used all the information we had, we had said all we had come to say.

Ushers collected the judges' ballots and carried them, like bank notes, to the chairman. The buzzing stopped as he opened the first envelope and extracted a white slip of paper. He put it on the lectern, to one side; ages later, it seemed, he located another slip, and finally the third; he added them to the pile. He still had his own little speech to make, thanking one and all, expressing his relief that *he* hadn't had to judge the debate, it was that close; and then came the skyrocket; by a vote of three to zero, the decision went to us. The applause was like thunder, cracking and crackling again and again.

We were bumped off in the next round by practically nobody, but no matter; we had seen the glory from the top of the mountain. . . .

Everything considered, small-town pupils were exposed to a fair amount of classroom and public appearance. . . . Grade school programs on Friday afternoons gave an opportunity to recite poems and other selections and to take part in short skits, before peers, plus a few visitors. In high school both junior and senior classes gave three-act plays at a local church or theater.

. . High-school assembly programs also often featured debates, readings, skits, and an occasional mock trial.[4]

We still had a ways to go, but so also did our teachers. In the first twenty volumes of *The Quarterly Journal of Speech* are frequent articles about qualifications for debate judges, criteria of good debating, and the importance of ethical standards. So while the founding fathers and their contemporaries were busily uplifting debate and speech contests, here I was in northwest Missouri lousing up the system.

WHEN SMALL TOWNS began to decline, Father and Mother bought a larger newspaper in Osceola, Iowa. I was graduated from Osceola High School and later from Grinnell College, and got a job (i.e. accepted a position) teaching English, speech, and journalism in the high school at Vermillion, South Dakota. I had thought of this move as a temporary, just-for-fun adventure, but during the first year I found I was enjoying my classes so much I abandoned plans for a newspaper career and contemplated becoming a professor of English.

I decided to go to summer school at the University of Chicago, perhaps because I had spent the summer of my junior year there, running a Linotype on the famous Printers' Row on South Dearborn Street and generally enjoying my first experiences in a big city. I had two brilliant professors, one in Anglo-Saxon and one in Shakespeare, and their assignments gave me a chance to get acquainted with the apparently endless resources of the University's vast research library. During my second year at Vermillion, however, I realized my interest in speech was even stronger than that in English. At that time only six universities offered a doctoral degree in speech. I might, for example, have considered Michigan, Northwestern, Cornell, Wisconsin, or Columbia, but decided in favor of the University of Iowa for a highly logical reason: my college schoolmate and girl friend, Augusta Towner (Gus), was teaching in an Iowa high school. Another reason, if one is needed, was that Iowa was one of the first two universities to be approved for the doctorate in speech, the other being the University of Wisconsin. On a visit to the Grinnell campus, Charles H. Woolbert, one of the aforementioned founding fathers, who had recently moved from the University of Illinois to the University of Iowa, had talked to our Grinnell debate club, mentioning that it was now possible to get a Ph.D. at Iowa, and had invited us to undertake graduate study in his department. I remember him as being of average height, friendly, relaxed, interested in young people, interested in his subject. He was then 50. He died a few days before I reached the Iowa campus.

In *Finally It's Friday*, I describe the experience of enrolling for a Ph.D. in this new discipline:

I had had no correspondence with the Department of Speech and Dramatic Art. I have since met graduate students in speech and history who were preceded to Iowa by glowing letters from presidents and deans, who were warmly received by their department heads, taken to see the graduate dean and other luminaries, and cordially welcomed into the company of scholars.

At the University of Chicago, the admissions officer had moved me, when he found I was a graduate of Grinnell, from the end of a long line to a short one. Right away I had felt like a special person. Here my experience was different. Here I was given the impression that only after careful scrutiny would I be allowed to join any line at all.

I was a real walk-on.

Now, in June 1929, I found myself in the office of E.C. Mabie, head of the department, to register for summer school. Mabie, short, stout, and volatile, whose disposition is better described by adjectives such as stormy, hard-driving, temperamental, and impatient, than by sweet and docile, lost no time coming to the point when I told him I was there to study for a Ph.D.

"How long are you going to stay?" he demanded.

"Until I get the degree. Three years or whatever."

"What speech courses do you plan to take?"

"Sooner or later, all of them."

"What is your main interest?"

"Public speaking and debating."

I had the feeling that one wrong answer, and I would be out in the hall. So far I had survived, simply because in my own mind, my purpose was clear. . . .

The inquisition continued. "Well, then, what courses do you plan to take now?"

Would there be no end to this barrage? this show of fire power? I had, however, studied the summer schedule. "Teaching of Speech, Advanced Public Speaking, and Discussion and Debate." I wondered from what direction the next shot would come. I did not have long to wait.

"Instead of Teaching of Speech," he said, "take Phonetics. Instead of Advanced Public Speaking, take Anatomy of the Vocal Organs. You can keep Discussion and Debate."[5]

NEXT MORNING I showed up in the auditorium of the Physics Building for the class in Phonetics, taught by a visiting professor, Stephen Jones, supervisor of the Phonetics Laboratory of the University of London. Jones had an easy, friendly approach to the subject and his explanations of the sounds that make up the English language were clear and stimulating. He did what a teacher should do: introduce the student to a field and encourage him to explore it further. Phonetics proved to be a prelude to courses in speech pathology, and also eventually led to my teaching phonetics for many years.

Anatomy of the Vocal Organs was taught by Henry James Prentiss, head of the Department of Histology and Embryology; the class met in an amphitheater in the School of Medicine, students sitting in elevated tiers, looking down on charts, specimens, and, occasionally, a cadaver. Prentiss was a master of dramatic exposition, aided by the widest assortment of charts and pictures and objects I have ever seen in a classroom. I readily developed a strong desire to learn how chest and stomach muscles, lungs and tubes and sinuses, tongue and lips and teeth, operated to produce human speech. Again, the interest aroused in that class persisted. Later, at Missouri, with the permission of the head of the Department of Anatomy, I studied the remains of what was once a human being, checking his muscles with the pictures in the manual, feeling the fibers to see where they began and ended, occasionally seeking help from the woman working at the next table, and in general tracing the sequence of events that lead to the production of human speech. I could not help wondering who my cadaver was, and what he did when he was alive, and how he happened to be here. Michelangelo once studied corpses, illegally and boldly robbing graves in the dead of night, studying the body's underlying muscles to see what shaped the texture of the skin, so that he could fashion a statue with greater naturalness. (It is comforting to be bracketed with Michelangelo, even in a small way.)

In the course on Debating and Discussion with A. Craig Baird I was on familiar ground. And when the six-week term was over, I stayed on for the second, five-week term. Most professors went on vacation, but one who remained was Harry G. Barnes. I was thoroughly fascinated by his course in Directing; I learned to view a theatrical production with an extra set of eyes, those of the director, and before long I saw I could watch a play and say to myself, "Now this nice bit happens because of the art of the actor, but this mood or effect or tempo is created because of the art of the director." I did not take any more courses in theater, but I did, during the two years that followed, and despite my heavy schedule, often watch Vance Morton or B. Iden Payne, a visiting director from the University of Texas, rehearse a play, and would become totally absorbed in noticing how they used stage areas and movement and timing to heighten the dramatist's concept.

So it happened that my first two summer sessions, one at Chicago and one at Iowa, opened whole new worlds of enchantment. At the time I would have said they were interesting because of the parade of new and different facts, but years later I would say to myself: At Chicago I learned to exploit the resources of a large library, a priceless gift in itself, to be treasured long after I had forgotten the facts of Shakespeare's sources or the nuances of Anglo-Saxon grammar. And during that record-hot 1929 Iowa summer I learned different ways of listening: to the sounds that make up language, with a deeper understanding of the muscles that produced the sounds, and to the ways of presenting the thoughts and emotions that make up drama.

So again: although part of a teacher's (an inside person's) mission is to impart an amount of hard fact, though much will be forgotten, another part is to make sure that a residue of discernment and insight will survive and prevail. The answer to "what did you learn in that course" is vastly different from the answer to "what did you learn today."

ONE AUGUST 1929 DAY I realized that the money I had saved from two years of high school teaching would not finance my stay in Iowa City "until I get the degree." Besides, my social life, so uneventful compared with that of undergraduate days, left chunks of empty time. I went to the *Daily Iowan*, the University morning newspaper, hunted up the Linotype foreman, Fred Flack, and inquired if he had a vacancy on the night shift. The fact that I was machinist as well as operator caught his attention; if I could make the repairs and adjustments necessary to keep his battery of four machines going, he would not have to make so many trips back at night to fix them. He signed me up for an eight-hour shift, 5:00 p.m. to 1:30 a.m., which meant I would be a student during the day, learning amazing facts about Greek rhetoricians and German psychologists, and a Linotype operator during the night, setting stories about the big stock market boom that was slowly making its way to the October date that in itself would be heavy drama.

In June 1930 I received my master's degree. Since I had previously passed the French examination, the committee could admit me as a candidate for the doctorate and advised me to start preparations for the German examination. In the commencement procession was W. Norwood Brigance, the first to get a Ph.D. in speech from Iowa, and by no means a walk-on, and Floyd Lambertson, an even older student also with years of college teaching experience. And though I did not know it at the time, Elmer Ellis, later to become president of the University of Missouri, received a doctorate in history on that day.

Gus was in the audience and after the ceremony we talked more earnestly than we had previously. A year earlier I had said it would be nice for us to get married when I got the Ph.D. and had a good job and a thousand dollars in the bank. Gus, at that time looking forward to another year of teaching English, agreed. Now I felt differently about the matter. We had corresponded regularly, and though I enjoy writing letters, I would sometimes reflect that with the time I spent writing her I could write half of a dissertation. I pick up the conversation from *Finally It's Friday*:

> She was thoroughly enjoying her second year of teaching. She was immersed in her favorite subject, English. She talked of going back, so she could have another year at the same school. Yet we wanted to be together.
> "You haven't finished your Ph.D.," she observed.
> "No. And it may take longer than I think. If I ever get it."
> "Once you said we should wait until you got a good job."
> "That's true. And right now the job market is tightening up."
> "You wanted to have a thousand dollars in the bank. How much do you have?"
> "Three hundred and twenty dollars and fifty-eight cents."
> She smiled. "I guess that's close enough."
> The girls have more courage than the fellows. She agreed to resign her job, much as she loved it, and move in on my three hundred.
> I suggested a June date. "No, I have a summer playground job. I'll need to get my clothes ready. But we can get married in August, after summer school." And then she added: "By then you'll have your German out of the way."
> As her offer was the best deal I was likely to make, I left it at that.[6]

The summer went rapidly; days in class, nights pounding a Linotype keyboard. The last Thursday afternoon in August I passed the required German exam; Friday I wrote course examinations; Friday night I went to Osceola to scrape a wardrobe of sorts together, and Saturday to Des Moines, where next evening we were married and drove away in the moonlight to honeymoon at Lake Okoboji.

IN SEPTEMBER, when I talked to Mabie at registration, he exploded another bomb; I should have a major in psychology as well as in speech. Here I was, with unusual preparation in English and history, ready to go ahead with the sort of study I had started at Chicago. I explained this, adding that I had had only a single course in beginning psychology. Hardly listening, he commented that I couldn't waste time taking beginning courses, but should head for graduate courses and seminars, and signed me up for a program including systematic psychology, abnormal psychology, physiological psychology, plus acoustics, plus speech pathology, plus assorted labs and clinics. Along the way, however, were seminars in literary criticism and British history where at least I had a fragment of background.

I survived mainly because I had developed investigative skills, maybe going back to the *Gilman City Guide*, maybe initiated in English and speech classes at Grinnell, maybe honed at Chicago.

Besides Baird, I had formed warm friendships with two Grinnell alumni, Barnes, already mentioned, and H. Clay Harshbarger, just beginning a career at the University of Iowa that began with the teaching of classical rhetoric, that proceeded to developing a program in radio broadcasting, and that ended as department head. Our small group talked politics and listened to radio programs—1930 was a year for much political speaking, and radios were now commonplace. Through communication the nation was becoming more closely knit. Anybody could buy a four-tube Atwater-Kent radio for $27.50 or shoot the works and own a ten-tube set for $150.

After the November elections, our conversation turned to the upcoming convention of the National Association of Teachers of Speech, the new name for the National Association of Academic Teachers of Public Speaking. Now in its sixteenth year, it had continuously printed a journal, stimulated research, and staged annual meetings that attracted not just 60 or 80 but four or five hundred teachers of public speaking and rhetoric, drama, speech pathology, and radio broadcasting. A fair amount of job hustling also took place; no scheduled system of interviewing was available, but professors learned from one another who was looking for what, and thus could alert graduate students who needed a job. Old-line publishers like Harper, Century, and Appleton, awake to the growing discipline, sent top people to staff their exhibits and to sponsor cocktail parties, all of which built almost as much name-recognition as their textbooks. Publishers were truly lovable in those days—they not only entertained you but gave you loads of desk copies, and if they had had good luck in merchandising your beginning text, they would publish your scholarly monograph even knowing they had small chance of breaking even on it.

When I learned that the Association was to meet in 1930 in Chicago, one of my favorite cities, and at The Stevens, the world's largest hotel, I was eager to go. I wanted to meet the people I had heard about, whose books and articles I had read.

Everybody remembers his or her first large convention whether he or she is a teacher, a merchant, or a Methodist. On the first morning, in the lobby of The Stevens, I saw, striding down a corridor, three huge men: six feet tall, broad-shouldered, bulky. I asked a stranger, "Who are those big fellows?" He laughed and said, "They *are* big fellows, in more ways than one. They are James M. O'Neill, James A. Winans, and Frank Rarig, three of the Founding Fathers of this Association."

If their names seem unfamiliar, think of them as Matthew, Mark, and Luke. O'Neill was the first president of the Association and also the first editor of *The Quarterly Journal of Public Speaking*, and department head successively at the University of Wisconsin, the University of Michigan, and Brooklyn College. Winans taught at Cornell University and later at Dartmouth College, and wrote one of the four or five most successful texts ever written for the beginning course in speech. At Dartmouth he became interested in Daniel Webster, and wrote a book about Webster's famous murder case. Rarig was for thirty years or more head of the Department of Speech at the University of Minnesota. On that campus a fine theater building is named for him. Winans and Rarig, after retirement, taught at the University of Missouri-Columbia, so a large group of our students had a chance to study with them. O'Neill, Winans, Rarig and a few others formed the first old-boy network and practically ran the Association for a quarter of a century. I could never have dreamed that many of the young teachers of my day would have met them and most of the other founders; and not only met them, but shared shop talk with them. These marvels are commonplace when a discipline is young. Right now I could only turn my head and stare until they disappeared into an elevator.

Later I saw, standing alone, a slender, graying man whom I recognized as the author of the text on parliamentary procedure that I was using. I straightened my badge and introduced myself in my clearest, most distinct tones. We chatted amiably, mostly about his book. When we parted, he said: "It's been a pleasure to meet you, Mr. Smith." I was so flattered by this personal attention I almost changed my name to Smith on the spot. Later, I mused, every young person has to wage a battle against Mr. Smith.

Another development that graduate students in the 1930s became aware of was that new Departments of Speech were being spun off from Departments of English. Here and there on college campuses radio broadcasting studios appeared, and speech clinics; often these activities were approved more readily in Departments of Speech than in Departments of English. A course in broadcasting or one in stage design might seem too vocational to a professor of literature.

Campus developments like these echoed what was happening in the general field of communication. In the White House, Roosevelt was eloquently showing the power of the spoken word in leading the nation out of the depression. In the 1932 campaign he brilliantly demonstrated the influence of radio speaking. His fireside chats from the White House attracted audiences of a size that other able speakers, like Bryan and Wilson, could not have amassed in a lifetime of face-to-face speaking. Through communication the nation was becoming more closely knit.

THE TOPIC I HAD SELECTED as my research topic was to write a study of the career of the English parliamentary debater and liberal, Charles James Fox. Few have excelled him in argumentative skill. He lived during the American and French revolutions, and supported both, despite heavy criticism, on and off the floor of the House of Commons. He bitterly fought the slave trade at a time when most people, partly for economic reasons, condoned it. He believed in freedom of speech and freedom of worship. I had written my master's thesis on Fox and received formal approval to continue with this topic toward the doctorate. The two or three biographies that had been written up to that time had offered little insight into Fox's abilities as a speaker. I had to fill in the picture by consulting numerous 18th century sources: correspondence, autobiographies, and newspapers. The interlibrary loan librarian borrowed books from over the country and I also found the Newberry Library at Chicago of immense help.

Then came weeks of digesting, analyzing, outlining, and writing. Finally I got the dissertation written and neatly typed on the required 20-pound bond. At the last minute the dean of the graduate school decided not to accept it, despite its having been approved by my adviser and by professors in major and minor fields. He said he had been a dean a long time and "just knew" what was and what was not a dissertation. I would have to rewrite it.

SOMEHOW, DISCOURAGED, depressed, drained, I got through 1931's torrid summer. At times I riffled the pages of the dissertation but could not summon the stamina to start a revision. As I analyzed the problem I began to see its two facets: the revision must be much shorter; the chapter headings and subheadings must display the word *speech* frequently so that even a graduate dean would see the focus. I wrote uncomplicated chapter titles like "The Speech of November 22, 1778," and subheadings like "Organization of the Speech," "Circumstances Under Which the Speech Was Delivered," and "Conclusions." Numerous one-sentence paragraphs kept the analysis up front, out in the open. Surely any one glancing through its pages would "just know" it was a dissertation in the field of speech. (Actually the 1778 speech was magnificent, powerful, so penetrating in its analysis that when Fox sat down, no one could think of anything to say by way of reply, and deserved better than routine analysis. A chapter about it deserved a more descriptive title than "The Speech of November 22, 1778.")

After completing the manuscript, I decided that, rather than retyping it, I would take it to the family newspaper office, now in West Des Moines, set it up on the Linotype and print it. It became a neat paperback of 124 pages. The day before the final examination I gave each member of the examining committee a copy, and deposited 35 copies with the University librarian, as required. The examination was set for July 14, Bastille Day, which seemed appropriate, in the House Chamber of the Old Capitol, the showpiece of Iowa's campus. As there was no air conditioning, the air was hot and oppressive. I sat at the long, wide, polished table, facing the six professors representing the graduate faculty. I expected a two-hour ordeal; I had spent weeks reviewing every course, anticipating every possible question. After twenty minutes, however, some one muttered, "Move we approve the candidate," and the vote was quickly taken.

The dean grumbled that I had not been given the full two-hour treatment; furthermore, he sent a circular letter admonishing the faculty to maintain the two-hour standard. But to my knowledge, he did not hold up any more dissertations in speech.

Charles James Fox, with 35 copies in the library, was readily available source material for graduate seminars. Its merits and its faults were clearly discernible. For a while it served as a kind of guide to the critical study of public speaking.

Now I return to the summer of 1932 [I write in *Finally It's Friday*]. Commencement was an outdoor, evening ceremony. The heat wave had broken; the sky was clear. With thirty others I stood in rented cap and gown to receive the blue and gold hood of an Iowa Ph.D. We were lined up in pairs, in alphabetical order. Next to me was a speech colleague, Herold Ross, of Depauw. He had also survived a rumble with the graduate dean.

As we quietly stood, a candidate broke ranks and walked to the head of the file. "What subject are you getting your Ph.D. in?" she asked Number 1.

"History."

"Well, I got mine in psychology. I worked harder for my degree than you did."

Before he could retort, she had addressed Number 2. "Economics." Again: "I worked harder than you did."

Others were from botany, biochemistry, experimental physics, English language, French. The inquirer had obviously been around a long time, had survived much torment, and had died a little in the surviving. To each her answer was positive: "I worked harder than you did."

She came closer and closer to where I was standing. "What did you get your degree in?" She hurled the words at me.

I looked her straight in the eye. I, too, had survived torment and had died a little in the surviving. "Speech."

She reflected, but only a second. "You worked harder than I did."

In minutes we heard the stentorian voice of Benjamin Franklin Shambaugh, Professor of Political Science, Introducer of Visiting Lecturers, Grand Marshal of Commencement, head and shoulders well visible above the potted palms with which the temporary platform was decorated. . . . Always the Ph.D.'s are conferred last of all, the climax of the program, the tribute to a centuries-old tradition. I can still hear him: "And now . . . will the candidates . . . for the degree . . . Doc-tor of Phil-os-o-phy . . . please rise."

Seventy-six trombones could not have done it better.[7]

Doctorates in speech (including theater and speech pathology) began to increase in number. At the end of the summer the department at Iowa had granted seven Ph.D.'s. In the whole country there were 33. Three years later there were, country-wide, 48, one for every state.

SELDOM DID A YOUNG COUPLE have a moment so dazzling, a future so uncertain. I could stay at the University of Iowa as a teaching assistant, but beyond that nobody knew what to expect.

Rossum's Universal Robots

HERE WAS THE SITUATION. I had resigned my high school position in South Dakota and, later, Gus hers in Iowa. After marriage we entered graduate school, so that eventually we could teach in a university. Within a year the Great Depression had arrived. In 1932 we learned of only one opening for a speech teacher in the entire country, at $2,000—considerably less than the once-prevailing, handsome salary of $3,500 for an assistant professor. We also overlooked another consequence: as a married woman Gus would find it next to impossible to get employment. The Great Depression had said: If you hire a woman whose husband is working, and so put two salaries in one family, you leave some other family without a breadwinner. It did make sense.

Older graduate students—in any field—who were on leave of absence, would have a position to return to, but younger graduate students had no such safety net.

As a university teaching assistant I had commiserated with my undergraduate students: the straight A senior engineer who said he would now have to go back to the family farm and milk nineteen cows every morning, the mathematics major who felt lucky that she had been offered a part-time bookkeeping job in the home town lumber yard, the brilliant young violinist who watched the opportunities in the musical world collapse and would have to postpone marriage until he found some other career. Conditions had changed as suddenly as that.

(Decades later I met that engineer. He said: "Do you know what I remember most about the depression? the bitter memory that won't go away? Milking nineteen cows.")

When, one day in 1932, now with a Ph.D., I learned of an opening in a high school, I leaped eagerly at it, especially since it was in Kansas City, the Big City of my northwest Missouri childhood. I entered this splendid metropolis riding the mighty Rock Island. I was interviewed by Superintendent George Melcher, who asked all manner of questions about graduate study and previous experience; he was relieved to know that I had already taught in a high school. "Did you have trouble with discipline?" he ventured; I could assure him that I didn't. An even more critical question was when he inquired whether I could direct a high school play. Suddenly I felt that my destiny as a teacher depended on my answer. I said simply, "Oh, sure," and held my breath awaiting his next move. He could have, but didn't, probe any deeper. Melcher's next question was whether I could start at midyear—it was then early in January—and when I told him I could, he offered me the position. Internally, I was jubilant. Even when he added, "Of course since we're now retrenching we'll have to cut your salary 10 percent next fall," I smiled like a busted watermelon, relieved it would be no worse. He assured me that his teachers would be paid, on time, each month. Everywhere schools were delaying paychecks, or tendering IOU's that were difficult to negotiate. Our group of graduate students had heard all the horror stories.

The proposed $2,000 salary for the spring semester, to retreat to $1,800 in the fall, was at the bottom of the Kansas City scale; the superintendent, faced with a budget crisis, had had to fill the vacancy in speech as cheaply as possible. (The top salary was labeled casually in the annual reports as "$3,000 and up.") If the opening had been in a traditional subject, he could have filled it within the system, but local talent was not available, and he wanted to maintain the school's active speech and drama program.

Westport, second largest of Kansas City's eight senior high schools, a few minutes by street car from downtown, was a proud school with many claims to distinction. It was the second oldest high school in Missouri, founded in 1852 in the nearby river port town of Westport; several of its teachers had master's degrees, at a time when advanced degrees were rare among high school teachers; its graduates enrolled in prestigious colleges. Probably no other high school, it claimed, had graduated so many Rhodes scholars. Sometimes it made the claim without the "probably."

Since I had been hired on short notice, I had conferred only briefly with Principal D. H. Holloway but I liked him from the outset: tall, balding, sixtyish, friendly. Our conversations were usually brief and businesslike but once he told me he had come to Kansas City from Boise, a community that still held his affection. "I wish I had my Boise job and my Kansas City salary," he said, wistfully, a situation that is typical of life's trade-offs. Mark Twain had reacted to this same dilemma when he said he liked heaven for climate, hell for society.

Leaving Gus behind to pack, I plunged into teaching without having met the faculty. When I visited my assigned quarters in the basement, I saw I was starting literally at the bottom. There had been a shuffling of rooms at the death of my predecessor, Albert S. Humphrey, an admired teacher with years of service, a student and later a teacher at Emerson College, and I had inherited a room nobody else wanted. Not quite a dungeon, not quite a regular classroom either, it had small narrow windows that pierced the outside wall, and utility conduits that snaked up the corners and crept across the ceiling. On one side was the industrial arts department and across the hall the boiler room. I would have to compete with power saws and pounding steam pipes. On the other hand, speech and drama students are vocal, so it was not a bad arrangement; we could be as lively as we liked. On a fair day high school pupils acting in a play or debating a hot issue can out-trumpet a Sousaphone. I would not have to worry about disturbing my neighbors.

During my first free hour my curiosity led me to inspect the building. I was strolling down the first floor hall when an older teacher, severe and heavily assertive, accosted me.

"What are you doing running around the hall?" she demanded.

"I'm new, and I want to see what the building is like."

"Well, here at Westport we don't just roam the halls because we want to see what the building is like. We stay put where we are supposed to be."

Later I learned that I was the youngest member of the faculty by half a dozen years, and as I well knew, looked younger than I was. As disarmingly as I could, I intimated I was still learning the rules. She mumbled but made no move to report me to the principal or to have me detained after school, and continued her tour. As soon as she was out of sight, I moved to the upper floors to continue mine. Before the hour was out she came downstairs to my classroom, totally embarrassed: "I'm sorry I spoke as I did. I didn't know you were the new teacher." She could hardly be blamed; in those days there were few young teachers in big-city schools.

That first encounter was inauspicious but more was to come. At noon I walked home to report my experiences to Gus and to snatch a bite to eat. When I returned, two student monitors halted me at the entrance. "Where's your home lunch permit?"

"I didn't know I needed permission from anybody just to eat at home." Then, artlessly: "Where do I go to get a permit?" The girls decided they had done their full duty by issuing a warning, and let me pass. I had taken only a few steps when I overheard the voice of a third girl: "You idiots, you stopped the new speech teacher." I turned and waved; they grinned sheepishly; we kept the secret forever. Teachers, new or old, don't need a permit to eat lunch at home.

In later years I would read about inner-city schools in Kansas City and elsewhere operating with massive security: armed guards at the single permitted entrance, teachers apprehensive of pupils carrying weapons, everybody alert for drugs. What a different world it was then, with pupils minding the front door and elderly teachers patrolling the halls, and coming to the building early and late, comfortable and unhurried, for conferences, meetings, and rehearsals.

WESTPORT'S COURSES were classified as *solids* and *non-solids*, the latter including performing arts like music and art, and industrial arts like shop and domestic science, which presumably required little or no homework. A non-solid course carried only half as much credit as a solid.

I regret to say I started my Missouri career as a non-solid teacher.

Colleges and universities did not then accept credits in speech or other non-solids. They preferred stiff doses of mathematics, science, English, foreign language, and social studies; applicants could fill in only around the edges with speech, art, music, shop. Teachers of our ancient disciplines, however, took this indignity in stride, assigning homework like everybody else. How can you teach public speaking, for example, unless your young speakers have done their study and thinking before they come to class? Eventually we would persuade university faculties that the pursuit of communication was a valid part of the curriculum. No overwhelming demand ever existed for poorly communicated wisdom.

I had been assigned to teach one course in "expression," which turned out to be the oral interpretation of literature, and another that had been recently renamed from "elocution" to public speaking. So although Westport was beginning to move out of the Age of Elocution, with its nineteenth-century sonorous glamor, it had not fully abandoned it. The rest of my schedule consisted of sophomore English, which was mainly grammar and composition with snatches of literature.

I still think of my Westport colleagues as diligent workers. Frederick Irion, in his sixties, taught five classes daily in civics, requiring written work; after school he carried home the outpouring of his 150 pupils, spent a long evening correcting, and next day handed the lot back. Hazel Wheeland, in history, in her forties, was intelligent and witty. On her desk stacks of reports came and went. One of the oldest was Ada McLaughlin, also a history teacher. It was she who had stopped me in the hallway that first morning. Came a day when, at the end of a spring semester, she took her examination papers home, read each one, recorded grades, signed the tall stack of grade cards, prepared the year-end report, turned off the lights, went to bed, and died in her sleep. End of the year; grades computed; reports completed. People said: What a way to go. An ordered end to a busy life.

AT TIMES I felt I was competing with the ghost of my popular predecessor; occasionally students would suggest I was not doing things the way they were accustomed to. I needed to establish my own style, to explain my own aims, and so enlist students interested in that approach. Since my second hour was vacant, I proposed at a faculty meeting that I would be willing to visit the classes of those who had second-hour classes, give their pupils a reading and speaking exercise, and afterwards offer suggestions that would help them to participate better in class discussion. At the same time I could collect data for a paper analyzing the speech proficiencies of a large mid-American high school. Twenty teachers—English, science, mathematics, history, home economics, language—agreed to let me visit their classes. In all I listened to 600 pupils, making judgments, on a simple rating scale, of voice, articulation, language facility, organization of ideas, and content. As the students performed I occasionally offered a suggestion, mainly to help them overcome shyness, or to project more forcefully, or to look at their listeners instead of out of the window. I could tell that as the hour progressed the students were learning from one another and from my comments. At the end I offered advice about reciting and discussing in class, under the general heading of the importance of communication in the classroom and in later life. People got to know the new teacher and what he taught.

In later years I would have to bridge the gap between speech and English. Now I was bridging the gap between elocution and speech.

One way or another I survived the semester. On a mid-June day I received the new contract that showed I had been reappointed with the promised 10 percent salary cut. As the payroll had been set up so that our last checks were twice the usual monthly amount, I even felt a momentary surge of wealth, the first since the stock market crash.

WHEN THE FALL SEMESTER opened, I found that enrollments in speech had so increased that I could drop the teaching of sophomore English and instead could teach a full schedule of public speaking and expression. Actually I was learning that years of graduate study were barely enough to fortify me to teach those two courses. Still, teachers must never underestimate their ability to read, to study, to observe—in short, to learn.

In those days teachers of speech, like teachers in other fields, could not be specialists. First of all we had to be able to teach a second discipline, such as English, since few schools could employ a full-time speech teacher. And if I had been able to teach only public speaking, I would hardly have been employable. Even colleges could appoint full-time speech teachers only if they could teach a variety of related courses such as public speaking, oral interpretation, radio, dramatics, and speech pathology. Once installed, however, one could gradually build interest in one's primary specialties and eventually teach them full time.

The Westport syllabus of the sophomore class in expression specified units in reading aloud and in elementary acting; I had taught neither. In graduate school I had had Harry Barnes's course in directing and a single course in oral interpretation, from a visiting professor, Mary Agnes Doyle. She was associate director of Chicago's Goodman Theatre, and herself a talented character actress. I had told her I would like to learn techniques from the art of oral interpretation that would help me teach the art of speaking in public. Speakers had long since stopped memorizing speeches and were now reading from manuscripts, and, with the exception of Roosevelt, usually poorly.

Doyle was intrigued and invited me to enroll in her course. Daily we read short selections aloud—from Shakespeare, Keats, Shelley, Whitman, and others. She emphasized sincerity and understanding of content—"don't just blahst away," she admonished, in her elegant stage diction. "Know the meaning of what you're reading." She convinced us that artistic communication demanded arduous preparation. She made believers of us.

From this single, six-week class, I learned anew that poetry was meant to be read aloud. I had known this already, or thought I did; my college professors of English continually read to us. What Mary Agnes Doyle, did, however, was to indicate even subtler nuances, using the voice's full resources of inflection, shading, loudness-quietness, fast-slow, pauses. She high-lighted connotations that we hardly knew existed. Shakespeare's comic scenes, for example, became funnier, and drama in poems like "The Highwayman" became more exciting, than we had previously experienced. She introduced us to a wide variety of selections that had special possibilities for reading aloud: poems, informal essays, scenes from plays. Many of these titles found their way into my classes.

In public speaking classes I jettisoned the syllabus's conventional memorizing of famous orations and let pupils make short talks on topics close to their hearts. Though we heard innumerable talks on trite subjects, we gradually moved to meaningful topics. Good content includes specific instance, organization, selection, audience analysis, colorful language. Sometimes the hour's speeches were set up as an informal contest, with listeners voting on who had made the best talk and who had shown the most improvement: to the two chosen I presented a pencil, or a paperback thesaurus, with enough ceremonial language to heighten the occasion.

One year, seeking to revive interest in an annual public speaking contest, I decided to invite Westport alumni who had been active in speech and theater to return and see what was currently happening. Holloway was intrigued by the idea—any principal likes to keep his school in touch with the community—and he and the office staff came up with a list of names, to whom I addressed a rousing appeal to come back and see what was going on at their alma mater. They came and listened to the speeches; I asked one of them to preside and each of them to cast a ballot; in short, students and alumni were thoroughly pleased with each other. After the meeting nobody seemed in a hurry to leave.

Speech teachers tackle communication from many different directions. At times I planned and directed all-school assemblies; at other times I worked with pupils who had serious speech disorders. The world of communication was headed for unbelievable changes and here was the beginning of a new era of an art that goes back to the dawn of humankind.

ALL THESE MONTHS a time bomb had been slowly ticking away. Suddenly it exploded; I was reminded that I was to direct the next school play, as I had recklessly agreed to do during the original interview. I must say that many, many teachers of rhetoric and public address in my generation had to do something with dramatics in their earlier years.

Of the Kansas City high schools, Westport had the saddest physical equipment. Already I had heard classroom speeches deploring the school's lack of a stadium. As for theater facilities, its stage was small, with tiny offstage areas; its footlights and overhead lights had only two switch positions, on and off—no dimmers, no floodlights, no spotlights. Its two sets, interior and exterior, must have been installed when the building itself was opened in 1908.

I scanned play titles, read scripts, sought advice from Iowa City. I located copies of twenty or thirty titles from which I would make a selection. Our apartment was strewn with texts; Gus, of course, was wholly involved. I needed a play that was "director-friendly": one with good plot and action, strong characterization, and good parts for girls as well as boys. I did not want a play with much talk and little action, and I did not want to open with Shakespeare. I persuaded the principal to advance funds that would include a decent royalty, in that day, $50.00; so many non-royalty plays are pure junk. If this account sounds to you like a public speaking teacher getting ready to direct a play, you are interpreting the situation accurately.

Eventually I selected *R.U.R., Rossum's Universal Robots*, by the Czech dramatist, Karel Kapek. Whenever you see *robot*, you can think of Kapek's play, which made the word popular.[1] The play's gripping plot made the job of actors and director easier. I needed all the help I could get, and a good book was essential.

R.U.R. had three sets, a formidable challenge considering our equipment and our talents. At this juncture Gus became Technical Director, Designer, and Chief Expediter. She had studied at Iowa with Hunton Sellman and Arnold Gillette, two of the country's well-known names in stage lighting and stage design. For this play about mechanical beings that threatened to multiply and take over the earth, she built and painted "The Central Office of the Factory of Rossum's Universal Robots," "Helena's Drawing Room," and "A Laboratory."

About 200 students tried out for this melodrama that featured factory-built creatures that looked like human beings but could do only the list of tasks for which they were designed: to be soldiers or secretaries, for example. A secretary-robot would have different built-in skills from a soldier-robot. Some were males and some were females; obviously they could not reproduce as that would add to the cost and reduce the efficiency. And there were national robots as well as universal robots. Eventually the robots would wear out and would be sent to the stamping-mill, a kind of recycling process—also a kind of death. In one experiment the inventor, toying with the formula, developed a new-style robot with remarkably human feelings. Thus the stage was set for complications, a necessity for good drama. We selected a cast of seventeen and planned to present the show two nights.

At the first rehearsal I took firm hold of the situation, explaining that play production was serious business, requiring dedication and concentration; anyone who stepped on the stage must assume the assigned role and not drop out of it. The drama's illusion must not be broken, even during rehearsal. On stage, robots must act like robots; the Engineer General should act like an Engineer General and not like a shy sophomore. I had seen amateur productions in which actors took sly peeks at their friends in the audience, got rattled whenever something went wrong, or became Sally Anne the minute Madame Beaumarchais stopped speaking. If the General Manager of the robot factory, played by a remarkably fluent student, George Eblen, were dictating to his secretary, a robotess, and a third character failed to enter on cue, the General Manager was to keep dictating, improvising dialog as needed, until the stage manager located the delinquent and shoved him on stage. The players liked the idea and even relished the moments when they could ad lib. The natural hams stood out.

I had also noticed that even experienced directors often assumed multiple responsibilities of locating properties, doing makeup, and prompting—an overwhelming burden of detail—so I selected students to do these important tasks. I could oversee without having to run errands. The student stage manager became responsible for entrances and exits, offstage phone rings and revolver shots, and the general conduct of rehearsals. I located a sophomore who wanted to make a career of stage lighting and put him in charge.

Together we worked out the lighting chart; from then on the responsibility was his. Never doubt that young people of almost any age can learn to do almost anything that we take the trouble to teach them.

We rehearsed six weeks. Two weeks before the play, a committee of parents told Principal Holloway I was working the cast and crew so long that their home work was suffering. "You're entirely right," he agreed. "Give me a list of the parents who are concerned and I'll see that their boys or girls are relieved of further responsibilities in connection with the play." The parents mulled that over, but no list ever appeared. In fact, Holloway never even told me about the interview until long afterward. Few things delight a teacher more than the support of the principal, or, for that matter, of the parents. So many teachers have to labor without either.

Hitherto, publicity for school events had been limited to hanging posters in the hall, making announcements in assembly, and inserting notices in the *Westport Crier*. Our committee did much more; we planned an assembly program that included a scene from *R.U.R.*, to introduce the notion of robots. With a home moving picture camera we shot a film, with subtitles, of intriguing scenes, using Hollywood cliches: *stupendous, colossal, thrilling*. Students were surprised to see their friends on the silver screen. At noontime actors in costumes, bearing signs reading: "Girl Robot" and "Boy Robot" paraded the halls. We were subtle in our interpretations; the robots moved and talked with just the slightest suggestion of their having been fabricated. Interest steadily grew in the upcoming performance.

A week before opening night, full-blown cases of mumps erupted. That was an emergency no committee could handle. I could only hope. Then, on opening day, the school was hit by student demonstrations and protests. There was talk of a walkout. The students wanted a stadium, and, if possible, right now. The commotion was so bad that school was dismissed at noon of the day of our first performance. I wondered whether the demonstrators would disrupt our show, but was unwilling to postpone it. We had sidestepped the mumps; we would take our chances with the strikers.

That night the auditorium was packed. The mood was the same as that of any opening night; the audience, including the protestors, was eager to see the show. I was in the hall, hoping for the best, and eight o'clock came before I realized it. Suddenly lights dimmed; curtains opened; the show began. The General Manager of Rossum's robot factory dictated: "To E. E. McVicar and Son, Southampton, England. ...." The robot secretary bent over her notebook. I joined Gus at the back of the auditorium.

After the first act, I went backstage. "I hope you didn't mind our starting without you," said the stage manager. "We finished the makeup early and everybody was ready, so when 8:00 came, we pulled the curtain."

He was following his checklist as the crew was changing Gus's sets. The 90-pound sophomore was adjusting a spotlight. A makeup girl was brushing powder off the ingenue with a rabbit's foot. The sound effects boy was sitting alert with two pistols; he had always been afraid that one might jam, and he wanted another at hand. The prompter took a fresh grip on the page opening Act Two.

Of course I didn't mind. My part of the show was over. Now it belonged to the kids. The play had action for everybody: war between robots and humans, people being killed off by robot soldiers, robots doomed because the secret of their manufacture had been destroyed, the future of the universe resting upon the improved robots who had somewhat human feelings.

We had another packed house the following night. By Monday the walkout was forgotten. Perhaps the play, bringing students, teachers, and parents together, had helped renew the sense of pride in Westport. We still deserved better athletic facilities, but they were only part of the school. The real school was the feeling of working together.

All in all I directed three plays, enough to carry me through the depression to better times, and then I returned play production to the experts. I was so rushed, teaching 150 students a day, spending after-school hours rehearsing plays or assembly programs, working with debaters or contestants, helping a girl with birth-injured speech, sometimes feeling like a standard universal robot with parts wearing out that could not be replaced, only occasionally like an improved variety with hope of a future. Of course on other days everything came together and I would feel I would rather be at Westport than anywhere.

EARLIER THAT YEAR I had given a paper to the Missouri State Teachers Association convention in Kansas City about the speech needs and abilities of high school students, using data from the survey of Westport second-period classes. In the audience was Frederick M. Tisdel, dean of the College of Arts and Science of the University of Missouri, who was quietly looking for an instructor in speech. Before World War I he had joined the Department of English as a professor of elocution, but after a year had been made dean. He had also been one of the early members of the old National Association of Academic Teachers of Public Speaking, so he was one of what I have called the first generation of speech teachers. At the end of the program he introduced himself and we had a short visit. I did not then know the purpose of his being at the meeting and attached no particular significance to the conversation.

Late one afternoon that spring I was sitting in my classroom, recharging my drained batteries for the walk home. In came Bessie Gay Secrest, speech teacher from Southwest High School, who said that the possibility of a Missouri Association of Teachers of Speech was being discussed. "Missouri speech teachers," she explained, "are now a small division of the Missouri State Teachers Association; all we do is hold an annual two-hour program and elect officers. We should have a year-round group to study our curriculum problems and improve the accreditation of speech teachers. It is deplorable that a teacher who has had little or no college credit in speech or drama can teach a high school class and direct a play or a debate. It's not fair to our talented youngsters."

She displayed a sheet of paper which a dozen teachers had already signed, accepted $1 for dues, and left. She became the first president of the group that was later called the Speech and Theatre Association of Missouri.

Thus I was in on the birth of this statewide organization, initiated by a group of high school teachers. What I have written is typical of the movement sweeping across the country. At the time I did not realize how easy it was to become a founding father. Later I became editor of the new Association journal, which bore the unprepossessing title of *Speech News*. I should have been more imaginative; I could just as well have called it *Transcendental Communication* and so could have gone on to all kinds of glory. At the Association's Golden Anniversary Convention in 1982, nearly 200 teachers of speech and theater gathered to recall their past and to explore the current state of the art. Bessie Gay could never have dreamed how her sheet of names would have multiplied nor how the field would have expanded.

EVENTS MOVED RAPIDLY. I learned that the Central Missouri State Teachers' College at Warrensburg needed an instructor in English and speech for the summer session—another example of the English-speech relationship characteristic of the era. In an interview, the president described the job: three classes in freshman English and one in dramatics—four classes a day, five days a week—eleven-week term, salary $425. On that handsome stipend the three of us—a year-old daughter had joined our family—could live all summer without dipping into our savings.

Just as I was beginning to think he would hire me on the spot, he said: "I'm worried about the class in dramatics. We might not get sufficient enrollment and thus couldn't keep you busy. Instead, we could offer a course in Victorian literature, which, we feel sure, would make. I really must study our situation further and decide later what to do."

I felt as if I were back in Chicago, ten years earlier, a college sophomore, pounding the streets, looking for a Linotype job. Through the soles of weary feet, being turned down by one foreman after another, I had learned that an interviewee must push his qualifications to the limit.

I had come to a critical point in the interview. "I can also teach Victorian literature," I said. "My undergraduate major was English. I have had ten courses in literature." I took a deep breath. "You want to get this settled and so do I. Why don't you hire me now, and let me know later what you want me to teach?"

To my amazement, he agreed. I had added another page to the art of interviewing. And as it happened I did not teach Victorian literature, though that would have been a fascinating experience.

I had been on the campus a fortnight and was in a relaxed and happy mood when the president stopped me in the hall. "How many hours a week are you teaching?" he demanded, unexpectedly, sharply.

I gulped. I was meeting four classes daily and directing the summer play. "Twenty," I said. He scowled, as if that were not enough.

A week later he asked again: "How much are we paying you?" I told him. "We *are*?" he said, and wandered off. I was shaken. Reduced pay and sudden dismissals were typical of depressions. I confided my alarm to my department head, C. F. Martin, a man of poise, grace, and humor, who dismissed the idea: "I know the budget, and you're on it."

Midway through the summer session I had a letter from Dean Tisdel. Would I be interested in an appointment teaching speech in the Department of English, with the rank of instructor, at $2,000? After a long period of retrenchment, the University of Missouri, like the nation, was beginning to come out of the slough. Perhaps Roosevelt's New Deal, with its famous alphabetical agencies like PWA, WPA, FDIC, CCC, was helping to boost the country's morale.

Gus and I were not eager to leave Kansas City. What now seems like an obvious decision, then was burdened with pros and cons. After a $2,000 year at Westport, followed by a 10 percent cut, we had crept up to $2,100. For the coming fall we had been promised the regular $300 raise plus a $300 "supersalary," a merit raise tacked on by central administration. Surely it would be folly to leave $2,700 behind to accept $2,000, nearly a 30 percent cut. I wrote Craig Baird, who counseled: "Often it is difficult to move from high school to college except at a loss. Think where you would be ten years from now." At the University of Missouri, full professors could climb to as much as $4,500. We decided to accept. The Great Depression was still ruling our lives; we could make the move, but at a cost.

We had no chance to say goodbye to Westport colleagues, and left Kansas City with regret. We had enjoyed the big city, the repertory plays that came regularly from Broadway, the new Nelson art gallery that was acquiring exciting items, the evenings with Grinnell graduates who had also located in Kansas City. Decades later the character of public school teaching had changed, but if I were to recall a dozen peak moments from my early teaching I would visualize a last-hour public speaking class of thirty juniors and seniors, convening on a bright afternoon in late May. They had selected their best speakers, three boys and three girls, and had invited a history class to be their guests. The room was packed, some standing, some sitting on the floor. Commencement was a fortnight away. The speeches were thoughtful but lively, with serious moments, vivid moments, humorous moments, sentimental moments. After the last speech, the room was silent; the bell rang; nobody stirred. Little spurts of animated conversation erupted over the room, and then, gradually, the class dissolved.

The year was 1935. The students came from mid-American, middle-class families that had struggled through the Great Depression. They walked to school, thirty blocks more or less, streetcar fares being an unnecessary expense; and if there were as many as a dozen who drove, they parked on a side street along with the few faculty cars. Or they walked downtown, thirty blocks more or less, to a movie, feeling entirely comfortable about it. After they were graduated and were getting started in careers, war broke out and ninety percent of the boys went into the military, most of them enlisting; half of them became officers. One way or another most of the girls were involved as well.

The years hurried by, and memories of Westport were shunted aside by the rush of events. Then one day came a letter from a committee of that Class of 1935: Could we attend their fiftieth reunion? We did; 200 people were there, maybe more; we met thirty or forty former students. We had last seen them when they were eighteen, nineteen; now they were in their sixties, approaching the end of active careers. We said: We can see much of the young faces in the old. They said: You're our last surviving teacher.

There were solemn moments: the reading of the names of the twelve who had died in World War II, of others who had died later. There was a showing of the old *R.U.R.* movie, doubly touching because some of the actors, robots and humans alike, were no longer with us. But there were goofy prizes, and dancing. The evening was a tribute to their alma mater, and also to their own courage and resilience as members of a generation from whom so much had been demanded.

And if I were to make a list of the dozen years I most enjoyed teaching, I would include one or two from that fine institution, my last high school, that bore the name of a pioneer settlement on the bend of the Missouri river. Later when I taught classes in speech education, supervised practice teaching, and wrote

Teaching Speech, many examples, illustrations, and basic principles came from the Kansas City experience. It was there, too, that I began to go regularly to meetings of state teachers' associations, sometimes as rank-and-file member, sometimes as parliamentarian, and got involved with a state association concerned with the field of speech.

8

Elocution, Speech, and Shakespeare

BACK IN 1931, Walter Williams, founder of the world-famed School of Journalism at the University of Missouri, then president of the institution, had had to quiet rumors that the University would have to close for a month, or for a year, because of drastic curtailment of funds. Now, in 1935, people could declare confidently that the University, having survived the Great Depression, would be around a while longer.

With a new daughter and a slightly used '34 Chevy, we were happy to be a part of this rejuvenated future. After five semesters in a city high school and a summer in a teachers' college, we were beginning a new job, the kind for which we had studied in graduate school.

Columbia was then a modest burg of 15,000, barely larger than Moberly's 14,000 and not so large as the state capital's 22,000. We did not then realize its potential for growth; eventually it would become Missouri's sixth most populous city (100,000, counting environs) and pushing fifth, because of its university and two women's colleges and its location in the center of the state at the crossing of major highways. We thought Columbia would forever be miserably handicapped because it had missed being on the main-line Wabash between St. Louis and Kansas City and would have to be forever content with being on a 21-mile single-track spur; when the Air Age came, however, it was ready with an airport served by Ozark Airlines.

On the campuses, the fall semester was upon us. Bookstores had stocked texts, notebooks, slide rules, fountain pens, pennants of the Big Six, later Big 8, schools. In our apartment, suitcases and boxes had been emptied, and closets, drawers, shelves, and the icebox, filled. Coming up was the first day of a university career that might, with luck, last forever.

IN 1935 THE PRESIDENT of the University was Frederick A. Middlebush, the sixteenth man to hold that office. Middlebush occupied a barn-like suite in Jesse Hall. Since in those days a president regularly interviewed applicants, I had visited with him briefly. I was among the first score of people he hired. He was the focus of so much authority, and appeared so awesome, that I can hardly believe he was only 45 when I first met him. Even less, I can hardly believe I was once 30.

During that era, university presidents could leap over tall buildings at a single bound. Deans and department heads could also leap over tall buildings, but had to be a bit cautious around the chimneys.

Middlebush had just seen his first budget through the legislature. In the appropriation was an extra $500,000 for salaries, though the governor later snatched $60,000 of it back. I have a deep interest in that appropriation, since I was paid out of the part the governor did not need, as were a dozen other young faculty newcomers.

During the previous two years, the faculty had endured a 15 percent cut. Departments had had little or no money for office supplies and equipment. The pool of assistants, graders, and instructors had been reduced 40 percent. Now the curators and president hoped to get the school back on its feet. The state could draw on its new sales tax revenue, at first paid with one-mill tokens printed on milk-bottle caps, and also from new liquor taxes.

Stimulated by the inpouring of New Deal funds, construction was booming on campuses everywhere. You could hardly visit a campus without having to avoid cranes, bulldozers, ditches and tunnels, blocked sidewalks. Aided by a $1.4 million Public Works Administration grant, the University began to construct six new buildings, including a new wing for the library that was tabbed at $310,000, a modest cost; ordinary laborers could be hired for 40 cents an hour and union members for $1.10. In Columbia, this extravaganza of building was the most impressive since the Great Fire of 1892, the one that gave birth to Missouri's famous free-standing columns.

Elsewhere in Columbia, Stephens College started a four-story classroom building and a large stable and show ring. Stephens has always had a happy mix of women and horses. City voters authorized a new Lee School, a new Ridgeway School, a Jefferson Junior High School addition. And a new county jail housed the thieves and drunks, who had been pretty crowded in the old structure.

Enrollments were up. With the largest freshman class in its history, the University reported an enrollment of 4,200. These statistics were reflected in the traffic at the Wabash and Missouri-Kansas-Texas depots. Hundreds of students bearing suitcases, laundry bags, portable typewriters, tennis rackets and other equipment, swarmed off the long trains.

Around the nation, faculties were being rebuilt. The Missouri campus saw brand new faces in chemistry, philosophy, rural sociology, law, psychology, physical education, English, and intercollegiate athletics—a welcome sight after the steady erosion of talent the preceding four years. The long-starved English department was allotted the largest number of new appointments, including several instructors in freshman English. Its faculty then included three in speech: Wilbur Gilman, Donovan Rhynsburger, and Bower Aly. I came not as a replacement but as an addition, a sign of the growing interest in speech, and although I had held the Ph.D. three years, I had only the rank of instructor. A large part of the College of Arts and Science, along with the President, Dean, and Registrar, was housed in a single building: Jesse Hall. Professors of English, history, foreign language, art, and psychology officed there and taught in its many high-ceilinged, reverberating classrooms. On the east side was the auditorium, a gingerbread creation of old-time elegance, its curved mezzanine supported by numerous pedimented pillars. Theatergoers enjoyed its intimacy but avoided seats with an obstructed view.

Once a week the combined ROTC outfits held a parade on the Red Campus. Troops were already on the march in Europe, but, again, that was a long way off. Still, our generation had memories of World War I and knew that a situation could get out of hand.

ALTHOUGH PROFESSORS OF ELOCUTION were indifferently regarded on college campuses, most people believed they knew what elocution was: the study of voice, gesture, and facial expression. Less well known was the fact that elocutionists taught these bodily activities not merely for their own sake but to heighten the meaning of what was being said.

We successors to teachers of elocution—we who called ourselves teachers of speech—had more of a problem in establishing our identity. What was it we did? Many thought we were chiefly interested in vocabulary and other aspects of language. "Oh, you're a speech teacher," someone would say; "I'd better watch my grammar." Or pronunciation. This attitude seemed reasonable, since most speech teachers had majored in English and were teaching in high school or college departments of English. When people asked me what "speech" was, I often merely mentioned a few of our courses, like public speaking and debate. If they sought further information, I was ready and eager to supply it. We found much to admire in Roosevelt, Churchill, King, Helen Hayes, the Barrymores and others, not only in their vitality as displayed in vocal variety and facial expressiveness, but also, especially, in their evidence and reasoning, the clarity and vigor with which they communicated ideas and feelings, their credibility, character, and judgment.

Often one hears public officials over television and sees them staring fixedly at a manuscript while making a statement such as "I am absolutely opposed to an increase in the public debt." Or perhaps the speaker is a corporation executive who rivets eyes on his notes and says in a gray monotone, "I am delighted to report that income is up 15 percent." One would think that the official or the executive would look directly at the camera and utter the words with liveliness so that language, eyes, and voice would all suggest firmness in one example, delight in the other. When Roosevelt said, over radio or news reel, "This nation will endure as it has endured," or Churchill, "We will never surrender," listeners knew from voice and movements as well as from words that the speakers believed what they said.

Speech teachers are not alone in having an identity problem. My colleagues in agriculture insist there is more to their discipline than farming; professors of law argue that even though many students do not actually practice law, a legal education is in itself a fine thing; wizards in mathematics want people to know that they go beyond algebra and geometry. Bankers have spent much of my lifetime convincing patrons that they really want to lend money and that they are nice and friendly about it.

Speech as a teaching discipline began modestly but grew rapidly. By the 1930s we claimed perhaps 200 departments of speech, most of them one- or two-teacher sections at colleges like Grinnell, Wabash, Knox, or Hamilton, but half a dozen were full-fledged university departments offering undergraduate majors and also master's and doctor's degrees. Eventually the number of departments would explode to 2,600 and more. Tens of thousands of students would learn first-hand what "speech" (or "speech communication") is. A 1985 governmental survey found communication to be sixth in rate of growth among the 30 disciplines studied.[1]

In 1935 the University of Missouri, like most campuses, offered courses in speech through the Department of English. Similar situations existed in schools like Washington University, the University of Illinois, and innumerable others. Our speech staff of four joined an English staff of seven professors and eleven instructors. In department meetings we joined the seven who taught the courses in language, literature, and composition. Four of Us and seven of Them, therefore, formulated policy.

I do not want to give the impression that English and speech teachers were antagonists or even counter-irritants. Both groups were committed to improving communication in one form or another. Courses in theater seemed to be a normal and natural part of an English department, since play production was a cousin of dramatic literature. Oratory could be viewed as a literary form, comparable with the grander forms of prose. Public speaking was akin to written composition; both activities demanded suitable organization, vivid language, and logical thinking. It also helped that the backgrounds of speech teachers included courses in language, literature, and composition. Actually, we understood their problems better than they understood ours. Many of us had had undergraduate majors in English.

On the other hand, the two groups had marked differences. One was age. Our average age was 32; Theirs was over 50. Another was rank; our group included no full professors. We were born and educated in the twentieth century; They were born in the nineteenth century and were educated by men who dated back to the Civil War. We had studied Latin but had missed Greek; They had got the whole bundle. Other differences were that the enthusiasm of professors of literature did not extend to courses like stagecraft, which seemed to them mere carpentry. And so far They had not had to reckon with a strange area like speech pathology, although They had approved a course in "speech improvement." Radio had not yet become popular enough to be troublesome to Them, nor speech science; only after prolonged discussion had They agreed to spend $700 for a recording machine provided the dean's office paid for it.

Even so, oral communication had had a long tradition at the University. Shortly after the Civil War, John R. Scott had been appointed professor of elocution. He had written a book, *The Technic of the Speaking Voice*; the title indicates his specialty. He was still living in Columbia when Gilman, Aly, and Rhynsburger had begun their University careers. After he had retired in 1910, the Department of English had annexed the field of elocution, the courses being taught by a series of young men.

Gilman, Aly, and Rhynsburger had gained permission to sponsor a major and a master's degree "with emphasis in speech," a combination that included courses in speech but also four courses in literature, chosen from four different areas. One could get a degree in English with no speech, but if one wanted a degree in speech one was required to include the four courses in English. The mixed program was not popular with students who wanted to take speech and theater courses free of the requirement in literature; these students shunned Missouri and went to universities like Northwestern or Wisconsin or Cornell which had separate Departments of Speech. During the earlier period when many teachers of speech also taught English, the mixed English-speech degree seemed appropriate.

The speech-theater segment of the English department officed in a small room on the second floor of Jesse Hall, along with two student helpers who were paid 25 cents an hour to help with clerical details. This munificence was from the New Deal's National Youth Administration's work-study program. The four speech teachers were paid a total of less than $10,000 and the eighteen English teachers less than $50,000, even including their stamps, stationery, and mimeograph paper; so for $60,000, the price of a single professorial star half a century later, the University furnished 4,200 students instruction in writing, reading aloud, speaking, acting, debating - and language, criticism, and literary history from Beowulf and Chaucer to the present day.

THE MOST POPULAR undergraduate speech course was the sophomore-level course in public speaking. My schedule consisted of four three-hour sections—two-thirds of the department's entire offering of this course—with 15 enrolled in each section. Half a century later the number had grown to 40 or 50 sections, with 25 or more in each section, and with long waiting lists; of a total staff of 50, 20 or more taught this introductory course. Total University enrollment had increased six-fold; enrollment in speech had increased twelve-fold or more.

I led students through narrative, expository, and argumentative speaking, an approach that reflected the influence of my being originally an English major. Freshman English texts also had sections of narrative, expository, and argumentative composition. Half a century later this organization of the course was still common.

I liked the notion of teaching the different types of public speaking. The narrative speech, for example, demands detail, climax, pause and other aspects of timing. Narrative adds variety and sparkle and lets speaker and listener share their common exposure to the talents and frailties of humankind. It mixes humor, anticipation, complication, suspense, and the shared background of information that makes it possible to appreciate the point being made. It is fundamental to communication; one trying to convince another person may tell a story to clinch the argument. The importance of expository speaking—the ability to make an idea clear—and of argumentative or persuasive speaking—-are obvious.

A feature that gradually disappeared over the years was a two-week exposure to parliamentary procedure. Yet when in the 1960s students rebelled at University authority, enough parliamentary sense of fair play lingered among campus leaders so that when they called a mass meeting to argue their claims, they asked me to serve as parliamentarian. It was a wild occasion with yells and shouts and bullhorns, but our rebels had a shred of common sense and listened to moderate as well as to radical voices. "This is what your motion says," the parliamentarian would rule, borrowing a bullhorn from Long-Hair-With-Beard; "this is what a yes-vote will mean, and this is what a no-vote will mean." If the rebels decided to tear the University down brick by brick, they at least would do it by majority vote.

Our many individual conferences with students echoed the friendly tempo of the campus. We were like assistants in laboratories looking over the student's shoulder, and like instructors in English, reading a theme along with the author. Years later, W. C. Curtis, dean of the College, described teaching before World War I. In that decade many professors scheduled their classes two hours apart so that after one class they would be free to chat with students. On Sunday afternoons students often came to the home of a professor for tea; in Curtis's home they filled the living room and found seats on the stairway. Our relationship with students was almost as close.

In my four sections were half a dozen women students. At registration, male students, especially those in engineering or agriculture, who almost never saw a female in their classes, might implore: "Can I be put in a section where there is a girl?" Sometimes I could say, "Yes, you can have a Betty, a Barbara, or a Jane. Take your choice." And a female student would ask, shyly, "Will there be other girls in the class?" and sigh her relief if there would be at least one other. The proportion of women students in speech classes was to increase steadily, partly because women became more career minded and the vocational advantages of being able to speak well became more apparent.

College catalogs listed not only the members of the faculty but also offered information about them. A student could discover not only where his or her professor had earned degrees but also the date of first appointment to the institution and the date of attaining present rank. Gradually this interesting academic pedigree was scissored away. Currently if you want to learn the academic titles of your teachers and how they spell their names, the catalog is a great place to look, but it yields little further information. Some catalogs do not even reveal which teacher teaches which course.

I missed the youthful enthusiasm of high school students but liked teaching at the university level. My various assortment of classrooms—among the rock collections of the geology department in Swallow, or just under the gables on the top floor of Whitten, or in the decaying auditorium in Lathrop—-was little improvement over my basement room at Westport, but I did not worry about the surroundings. In four years, even with small classes, I taught the fundamentals of making an idea interesting to an audience to more than 400 young men and women, including a high percentage of out-of-state students who then paid no more tuition than the natives.

IN THOSE DECADES the notion of department "head" was well established. Once a head was appointed he (almost never she) served forever. He made the decisions and accepted the responsibility. The idea of a rotating chairperson who presided, rather than directed, was yet to come.

The head of the Department of English was Arthur Henry Rolph Fairchild, whose specialty was Shakespeare. I seldom if ever heard him called "Arthur." A catalog entry read: "English 135. SHAKESPEARE. Mr. FAIRCHILD." No course description. What could be beyond combining "Shakespeare" and "Fairchild"? Especially when the course was popular, with a large enrollment? As head, Fairchild was formidable. Staff meetings became grim when professors argued whose scholarship was superior. A topic such as apportioning a hundred dollars among half a dozen people for convention travel was treated with gravity; after token discussion the head announced his decision. Off the campus, however, the Fairchilds were genial hosts. A houseful of us enjoyed a superb buffet, and afterwards played games like "twenty questions" and treasure hunt.

At a staff meeting, Gilman proposed to establish a speech clinic, with me as director. I described what went on in a clinic, outlining a plan to work with students who were referred to it. Henry M. Belden, a former head of the department, thought the enterprise desirable, but his colleagues gave it little support.[2] Speech pathology and a clinic sounded more like a scientific than a humanistic endeavor, obviously out of place in a Department of English.

For a while nothing happened. Then at a staff meeting, Robert L. Ramsay, one of the three University professors with a beard, a genuine, established authority on Mark Twain and on Missouri place names, told the group that one of his good students had a bad speech habit.[3] "She was reading Milton—and—*er, ah*—repeatedly inserted a loud *er, ah*, just as I am—*er, ah* doing. And like this: 'Hence . . . *er, ah* . . . loathed melancholy . . . *er, ah* . . .

Of Cerebus . . . *er, ah* . . . and blackest midnight . . . *er, ah* . . . born

In Stygian . . . *er, ah* . . . cave forlorn . . .'

"I can't recommend her for a position in literature so long as she has that defect. If we had a speech clinic, could she get help with her problem?"

Fairchild looked to me for an answer.

"Yes, she could. We call this problem the 'vocalized pause' and know how to teach the student to manage it."

The upshot was that I conferred with Emily (to give her a name). As she read for me, her *er, ah*'s were as conspicuous as dandelions on a lawn. Obviously she had no idea she was inserting these extra sounds. I recorded her speech on the new machine we had just bought, so she could hear herself. I asked her to read a passage and deliberately insert *er, ah*'s and then attempt the passage and omit them. "If you want to pause, just pause. A pause can have meaning. A pause can be a form of eloquence. You don't need to fill the gap with sounds." After a few sessions she was convinced that she could show Ramsay that she could read properly. I also worked with her on the art of reading aloud: the phrasing, timing, voice modulation, and study of the passage necessary to reveal the richer meanings. I wanted to develop her latent talent. Reading poetry is more than eliminating vocalized pauses. Emily knew that her career was riding on my approval but especially on Ramsay's.

When Ramsay was able to tell his colleagues that Emily was "cured," they agreed to establish a speech clinic; the art and craft of speech pathology was now shown to be related to the art of literature.

In the 1930s the idea of a speech clinic was relatively new. James M. O'Neill, whom I have already introduced as a founding father of the national speech association, while at the University of Wisconsin, had been perhaps the first to introduce courses in speech pathology, along with a supporting unit where students could receive diagnosis and therapy. This unit he proposed to call a speech "clinic." The faculty of Wisconsin's medical college opposed the use of the word "clinic"; the term, they argued, was the property of the medical profession. O'Neill, never one to avoid controversy, stuck to his guns, and "clinic" came into the language with a broader meaning than the physicians wanted. Before long there were reading "clinics," writing "clinics," and even hog-raising or photography or traffic control "clinics."[4]

Professors in various University divisions referred students to our new clinic. A star pupil was a Tiger quarterback who so mumbled his signals that the players ran into each other instead of into the enemy. Another was a visiting professor from overseas whose English sounded like Old High German. We trained a small group of clinicians and held workshops in central Missouri schools. I also gave a report to the new Missouri Academy of Science. Soon the Department and the College approved supporting courses in speech therapy and pathology. In two years we were ranked by Consumers Research as one of the twenty best clinics in the country. The decision to establish a clinic was the most far-reaching the Department made the four years I was a member of it.

If You Love 'Em, Join 'Em

MY SENIORS in the speech corner of the Department of English had long been alert to problems that secondary school teachers had in teaching speech and directing extracurricular activities.

As a judge at drama festivals, Donovan Rhynsburger had seen inept presentations of talented high school students who had received dismal direction from English teachers with little experience in the theater. Wilbur Gilman and Bower Aly, when judging debate and declamation contests, had viewed innumerable flabby efforts at speaking that resulted from untrained teachers. A school that would not turn its football team over to "just anybody" often did exactly that to play casts or debate teams. Debate techniques of researching facts and organizing arguments logically are learned skills even more subtle than those of being a wide receiver. And acting not only requires as much bodily control as athletics but also demands sophisticated use of vocal nuances. Gilman, who taught the course in methods of teaching speech, knew the difficulties in certifying and licensing teachers of both English and speech. One who sought to teach and to direct extracurricular activities in speech and theater should have had the basic preparation.

The situation in Missouri capsuled a nation-wide problem.

As second president of The Missouri Association of Teachers of Speech, Gilman used his considerable administrative talent to strengthen the discipline by working through other educational groups. When the Missouri Academy of Science was organized, he persuaded it to include a section at which teachers of speech could discuss phonetics, speech pathology, and speech science. He appointed a committee to prepare a high school course of study, one of the first in the land; it reflected the increasing emphasis on speaking as communication rather than as performance. The new journal, *Speech News*, went not only to Association members but also to teachers of English who taught speech classes and to superintendents and principals, keeping schools informed about Association activities.

Gilman, Aly, and I went to Jefferson City to interview Lloyd W. King, State Superintendent of Education. We were there to speak not as individuals representing a single campus, but in behalf of our Association. The superintendent received us cordially and offered us cigars, not an unusual gesture in those days, and asked us to state our problem.

Gilman said that those who were licensed to teach speech should have academic qualifications in that discipline. King did not say, "Now what is this 'speech'?" or "Just what is it that you teach? You're really not an academic subject, are you?" What he did say was: "Of course. What qualifications do you suggest?"

We were prepared to offer arguments, but since he agreed, we did not present any at all. It's a good idea not to argue with some one who already agrees with you.

Gilman did say: "We urge that every classroom teacher of speech should have a basic course in each aspect of our discipline: public speaking and debate, dramatics and oral interpretation, speech pathology. We would like to see a teaching major with standards as high as those required for other areas."

King was interested: "Are you people pretty well agreed on this?" "Yes, we bring these recommendations as coming from our Association." King pushed a button and his secretary entered. "Eleanor, make a note to call a meeting of the staff to discuss qualifications for certifying new teachers of speech." Then to us: "What next?"

We continued: "We would like the State Department to add to its staff a state supervisor for speech. This individual would travel and conduct workshops." We knew that other fields had state supervisors. King pushed the button again. "Eleanor, remind me to take up the possibility of a speech supervisor at the meeting of deans of schools of education when they meet here next week." Then to us: "What else?"

Our surveys of the speech needs of Missouri pupils had shown that 10 percent had speech difficulties—a standard finding of that day. We mentioned this fact and continued: "We would like the state to provide a fund to help school districts appoint a speech pathologist to visit classrooms and identify pupils who stutter, lisp, mumble, or in other ways need specific help, and advise teachers and pupils about remedial exercises."

King again summoned his secretary. "Eleanor," he said, "take a law." He smiled at his own phrase and she smiled and the three of us smiled as he asked her to call a meeting of his legislative advisory committee.

We were there less than an hour. When we left we were so light-hearted that our Chevy probably made the homeward trip on a quart of gas. Eventually these recommendations were approved. The new law put a number of speech pathologists in Missouri's school districts. A supervisor, Raymond P. Kroggel, began traveling around Missouri, conducting workshops. The new requirements meant that Missouri pupils could have qualified teachers. The "non-solid" had jelled into, almost, a "solid."

This interview demonstrated that an organization can do things for its members that they cannot do for themselves, a principle long established by trade unions. What public or private school teachers out there, or what professors, really think they would be as well off as they are, if it were not for state, regional, and national associations?

Years later I learned another reason why our visit went so smoothly. The Kings had a daughter, Katherine, a student in the Jefferson City senior high school, who was participating in the speech program under a talented teacher, Agnes Rank. They were aware of the improvement in communication skills achieved by their daughter and her friends. Since the heart of any program is the teacher, our interview was successful largely because the ground had already been laid by a competent, respected classroom teacher. What we did was to get buttons pushed that were ready for pushing. There are people whose careers are focussed on their classes, and people who move into prominent academic groups, and although a certain amount of glamor is attached to developing a statewide or nation-wide reputation, the groundwork has to be laid by able, stimulating teachers like Agnes Rank and thousands of others. (Rank was a hard-working outside person as well as a talented inside person; she had been active in Missouri's speech association from its earliest days, and was well known across the state.)

AS A BRAND-NEW PH.D., I had heard in 1932 about a proposed association for the upper Mississippi Valley, including North and South Dakota, Nebraska, Kansas, Oklahoma, Minnesota, Iowa, Missouri, Wisconsin, Michigan, Illinois, Indiana, and Ohio. The immense industrial and agricultural territory of these thirteen states, if transported overseas, would cover most of Western Europe. Giles Wilkeson Gray, my professor in voice science, had invited what was then called the Federation of Central States Speech Associations to hold its first formal convention in Iowa City. As "federation" suggests, the group was composed of individual state speech associations. Alan H. Monroe, of Purdue University, the first president of the Federation, had recently (1929) been involved in the formation of the Indiana Association of Teachers of Speech, and had seen that the discipline's problems in Indiana were common to most states.[1]

The Federation met in the spring of 1933, concurrently with the Iowa Conference of Teachers of Speech. As many states had not yet organized—Missouri not until 1932—the "federation" concept was dropped in favor of a new title, Central States Speech Association.

The Association had made such a timid start, however, that it had held only two conventions its first five years—at Iowa and at Northwestern. Now, in April 1937, it was pulling itself together for a meeting on the campus of the University of Wisconsin, but the outlook for survival was so dubious that the final afternoon was to be reserved to discuss this disquieting issue: Should the Association be disbanded? broken up? rent asunder?

Since the Association looked moribund I did not attend the convention, and was surprised to receive a telegram from Madison, asking if I would serve as executive secretary of this feeble enterprise. Those at the convention, after much discussion, had voted to forge ahead. Here was a battered old dog, struggling for breath, eyes rolled back, tongue hanging out; see if you can revive him. The honor was short of being enthralling.

I telegraphed an acceptance, nevertheless, and awaited the consequences. In a few days the outgoing secretary sent me the fragmentary records that represented the material holdings of the Association. Money? there was no money.

That fall our local speech teachers—from the public schools, the two colleges, and the University— assembled to make plans for a 1938 convention in Columbia. We determined to plan a landmark event. We called our local group not simply a "Committee on Local Arrangements" but a "Conference Executive Committee"; Wesley Wiksell of Stephens College ran it, and few could have done better. The general directive was: spend what you need and eventually we'll pay the bill out of convention receipts. That's the formula under which mighty world fairs and Olympic games operate. The printing bill proved to be enormous—$200—a month's salary—for 8-page programs, stationery, postcards carrying the preliminary announcement. Heath Meriwether of Artcraft Press, later printer to the speech profession, did not trouble us for prompt payment.

We outlined a program featuring the best-known people in the field: the authors, the researchers, the good teachers. Our procedure was not at all like that of later years in which a global "call for papers" is extended to the rank and file, resulting in a high percentage of new faces and of studies-in-progress. We commissioned the top talent. The program we put together still reads like a who's who of the discipline: Frank M. Rarig (Minnesota), Wendell Johnson (Iowa), Lee Norvelle (Indiana), Daniel Webster (Dartmouth), W. M. Parrish (Illinois), Ralph Dennis (Northwestern), Alan H. Monroe (Purdue), A. C. Baird (Iowa), E. C. Buehler (Kansas), John C. Calhoun (Yale), Irving J. Lee (Northwestern).

I admit that two names in the foregoing are sleepers; I included them just to give your eyeballs a yank.

Tributes can and have been written about each name in that remarkable list. I choose one, almost at random: Irving J. Lee, remembered, like the others, by only the oldest among us. Born in New York City, Lee received his bachelor's degree in English, taught social studies in a high school for three years, received his graduate degrees in speech from Northwestern. A university does not often hire its own Ph.D.'s, but Northwestern was wise enough not to let him get away. His course introducing General Semantics was enthusiastically received by students from all divisions of the university. He became interested in the problem of communication in organizations, and spent a semester at Harvard Business School, where a "case study" method was being developed (this in 1951). I can hardly put a limit to Irving's versatility; requests for his services came from business, industry, and government; he gave a hundred, two hundred, three hundred or more lectures to all kinds of groups. You will probably find a couple of his books in your campus library. I liked him because, plus the above, he was lively, imaginative, friendly, humane. He died at the age of 45.[2]

WHEN THE NATIONAL ASSOCIATION met at Christmas time in Chicago, I made a two-minute speech at the convention luncheon to advertise our plans for our 1948 regional convention. I rang the changes on "Columbia, April 1 and 2." "If someone asks you where and when the Central States Speech Association meets, tell them: 'Columbia, April 1 and 2.' Never let go of those dates—April 1 and 2. Write them on the wall of your office—April 1 and 2." Then a couple of glamorous sentences about program features, followed by: "I do not want to sit down without telling you the dates—April 1 and 2—in Columbia." Listeners chuckled at this transparent use of the oldest of all rhetorical ploys—repetition. One knows little about communication until he or she learns about repetition and its first cousin, restatement.

Chance plays a role in human destiny, as the Greeks well knew. If a statue falls, said Aristotle, and kills the man next to you, but spares you, count it as a piece of good luck. If you are handsome and your brothers are homely, that also is a piece of good luck. Among the listeners that day was the head of the Department of English at Washington University, St. Louis, who was seeking a speech teacher. My announcement caught his ear, so when he returned home he wrote inquiring if I would be interested in an assistant professorship. The salary offered was $2,400, more than I was currently being paid.

Just before the interview I twisted an ankle, so I entered his office on crutches. He smiled and said, "Sprain your ankle? I've just sprained mine, too," and lifted his foot, in a plaster cast, and rested it on his desk. We talked about ankles and then, with no inquiry about my qualifications, he indicated that the position was mine if I wanted it. I replied that I was interested but wanted to consult my wife, and was soon on the train on the way back home.

Earlier that spring Dean Tisdel had said I was scheduled for a hundred dollar increase—"it's not much but maybe it will help a little." He also had explained that University policy required that teachers with similar experience needed to be paid similar stipends—if a professor in a certain bracket were increased $200, everybody in that bracket would need to be increased. He also repeated his philosophy that "the University of Missouri is a good place to come to and a good place to go from." The first time I had heard him say this, I thought it meant that after a year or two I would be fired. Gilman, however, said it meant simply that Missouri was a respectable place to be. "Still, we do seem to lose our good people after a time," he added, sadly.

Tisdel not only opposed jostling his salary schedule but in other ways had fortified himself against innovation. Once I had gone to him with a proposal to add a new course. "Why, that's ex-*pan*-sion!" he declared, pronouncing the word in a hushed tone much as he would a-*dult-ery*. I returned later with a modification; I was now teaching two sections of Course A and would combine them if I could teach one section of new Course B. As that suggestion did not sound like ex-*pan*-sion, he approved it.

When I showed him the offer from Washington University, he gulped but said: "We'll meet it." I thanked him but left his office puzzled; what had happened to the bracket theory? or the expansion theory? After an exchange of letters, Washington raised the ante another $300. I reported this development to the dean. He swallowed hard. "This is highway robbery," he said, between swallows. "It'll take forever to get my salary schedule tidied up. But—but I'll pay it."

Gus shared the weighty decision to stay. Already she had moved five times in seven years and did not relish packing the barrels again. More to the point, she was delighted with Columbia and had secured a position teaching public speaking at Christian College. We also reflected that in a fortnight we had received a substantial raise, and had caught up to what we would have received had we stayed at Westport High School. I had still another speculation: "What if I had declined to be executive secretary of the Central States Speech Association? I would not then have made the announcement at Chicago and thus might not have come to the attention of Washington University." Enough of that line of thought; one can go raving mad if he starts down the "what if" trail. If the statue misses you, don't worry about it. And not long afterward I became an assistant professor. Five years had passed since that hot summer evening I had received my Ph.D.

Back to the Columbia convention. On the evening of March 31, 1938, the Wabash Cannonball disgorged a trainload of teachers, who headed for the Tiger, Daniel Boone, and Ben Bolt hotels. On April 1 and 2, as advertised, the convention began. Switzler Hall had 300 delegates attending meetings in its classrooms. Each delegate had paid a convention fee of $1.25; the total sum was exactly enough to pay Artcraft Press and our other creditors. We ended the year as we began, with a zero-based budget. But from then on the Central States Speech Association thrived. The convention held in 1939 in Minneapolis again attracted 300.

In 1981 a thousand persons attended the golden anniversary convention in Chicago—most in their own cars over four-lane highways or by one of a dozen different airlines; hardly anybody by train. At any hour of the day people had a choice of eight or ten different programs. Three Switzler Halls side by side could not have handled the event.

The Missouri Association of Teachers of Speech also grew and thrived. Its early meetings had attracted only 25 or 30. Temptations to split into separate speech and drama groups were solved by adopting new policies and a new name: Speech and Theatre Association of Missouri (STAM). In 1982 it held its Golden Anniversary at Springfield, and I was invited to give the banquet speech. To the hundred or more gathered in the banquet room, I pointed with pride to the last fifty years, and painted a vision of the next fifty. I felt like Daniel Webster giving his oration at Bunker Hill in 1825, reviewing the growth of the young nation since the battle of 1775, becoming a nation of 24 states, and extending to the Mississippi. A banquet orator, any banquet orator, should do no less.

WE ARE TOLD our ancestors survived the challenges of the jungles and the savannahs because, among other characteristics, they developed refinements of communication that competitors in the animal world did not possess. Hunters could plan in advance how to kill the mammoth—discussing procedures, selecting weapons, assigning tasks. After the mammoth was killed they no doubt shouted or made satisfied noises, or laughed together about their close calls. They created narratives about the event. Back at the village they praised their bravest and presented him with a choice bit of loin meat from the carcass. They mourned the fate of one who got too close to the mammoth's tusks. They scolded the hunter who missed the hunt altogether because, not being a good listener, he failed to note the time and place of rendezvous. Maybe, amid yells and jeers, and because he was always behind, they presented him with a chunk of the tail. They talked shop for hours. (As for the mammoths, eventually they became extinct.)

Teachers and their families need people to talk to, professionally and socially. Lewis Thomas describes the reaction of listeners to the new ideas presented at a lecture: "As the audience flows out of the auditorium, there is the same jubilant descant, the great sound of crowded people explaining things to each other as fast as their minds will work."[3] Thomas describes himself as a "biology watcher," but he is also a "language watcher," writing more than one essay about the phenomenon of language, the origin of words, the drift of meanings, showing that speech is the membrane that holds our communal cells together, and without which we would simply fly apart.

5

Growth of a Discipline

ARISE of state-wide associations of teachers of speech in the 1920s and afterwards and the formation of Departments of Speech followed the founding in 1914 of the National Association of Academic Teachers of Public Speaking.

I tell this story about the growth of the discipline because I grew up with it. As a high school student I competed in oratorical contests and debates, sponsored by a league that swept up the winners of local contests into district, regional, and state events. I was an undergraduate in one of the first colleges to have a Department of Speech. As a beginning high school teacher I attended conventions of the South Dakota Teachers Association, including the sectional meetings for teachers of English and speech. As a graduate student I judged high school events, managed a state-wide contest for one-act plays, learned that there was such a thing as the Iowa Association of Teachers of Speech, and attended my first national convention.

Another reason I narrate the growth of the field of speech is that in recent years I have met young people who seemed to know little about anything in the discipline that happened before, say, 1975. I pick 1975 because it was, let's see, the year I retired.

Once I had a hearing test, administered by a businesslike audiologist. She seated me in a small outer room; through a window I could see the familiar testing equipment in the inner room. She asked questions and made checks on a form.

"I'm a speech teacher," I volunteered, wanting to learn more of this person who was about to reinstall marvelous ranges of frequencies in my hearing. "Speech teachers and speech pathologists used to go to the same conventions, so I got to know many people in your field." All this in my friendliest, let's-get-acquainted, patient-clinician, mode.

"Oh?" she said. "How nice. Now I'm going to play tones of different pitches and you'll hear them through these earphones. Gradually I'll reduce the volume. Whenever you hear a tone, lift your finger." She demonstrated the tones and the lifting of the finger. She wrapped two big earphones around my head. I pushed one of them to one side so I could continue the conversation. "You've heard of Dr. Robert West. He was co-author of that famous textbook, *The Rehabilitation of Speech*. I often met him at conventions."

I could have added, but didn't, that in England I had met British teachers of speech for whom *Rehabilitation* was *the* book to know.

"No, I'm sorry I haven't." Once more she cozied the earphones into their proper place, and with a slight lift of the eyebrow, a sort of transition between my world and hers, she explained the next test and retreated to the inner room.

How sad, I thought, not to have heard of Bob West—fine scholar, magnificent friend, mountain climber, bridge player. I settled down to the finger-lifting.

When she emerged, test scores in hand, I mentioned a scholar in her specialty who had spent a lifetime on the campus where she studied. "I've heard his name," she said, rustling her data. "There is an auditorium named after him. Or maybe an award or prize."

I came down another bundle of years to get to her decade. I dropped another name or two. She gave me a look that said would I please halt the chatter, sit up straight, and pay attention? "Now here are your test results," she said, setting me free from the earphones. "And now let's make your ear molds."

Well, yes, let's.

That evening she must have told her husband: "In this business you meet all sorts." That evening I reflected: Audiology, in fact, is a different specialty from speech pathology. I must remember this. Nowadays you can practice one without the other. I must remember this, also. And maybe it is not necessary to know about the people of an earlier day. Maybe it is not necessary to go beyond the manual. Everything that is necessary and usable has happened since 1975.

At speech conventions I have heard people pronounce Winans as "Winnans," and are stumped completely by Thonssen or Aly, and I wonder if they, too, are post-1975. (For the general enlightenment: "Win" as "wine," "Thon" as "tahn," "Aly" rhymes with "daily," not "dally.") Then there was the Louisiana State University professor, Giles Wilkeson Gray, editor, researcher, co-author of the far-ranging *The Bases of Speech*. At a convention a young man approached him, peered at his name tag, and exclaimed: "You're Giles—Wilkeson—Gray! I always thought you were three men!"

Cicero, philosopher and epistler as well as political and forensic orator, put it this way: "He who is ignorant of what happened before his birth is always a child." Surely that is as true in 1975 A.D. as it was in 75 B.C.

THE FIRST STATE SPEECH ASSOCIATION to be organized was the Iowa State Association of Teachers of Speech, in 1921. Others followed: Texas, 1923; Michigan and Wyoming, 1925; Ohio, 1926; Southern California, 1928; Indiana and Illinois, 1929; Alabama, 1930; Oklahoma and Oregon, 1931. The movement was slow, deliberate; it hatched about one association a year.

All of these state-wide groups were operating before the Speech Association of Missouri was organized in 1932. That year the State Association of Teachers of Speech in West Virginia got under way. In 1936 The Ohio Association of College Teachers of Speech had organized a separate group of secondary school teachers, with Central, Southwestern, and Eastern branches. One of its objectives was to go on record favoring a Department of Speech at Ohio State University; the department was established later that year. By 1940 state associations had been organized in Washington, New Jersey, North Dakota, South Dakota, Colorado, Pennsylvania, and Arkansas. The 1950 *Directory* lists 39 state groups. Four regional groups, Eastern, Southern, Western, Central, were well under way.[1]

Inevitably, associations had a strong interest in the public schools. A statement by the Ohio Association of Secondary Teachers of Speech cited these goals: All high schools should offer speech courses. Ohio colleges should recognize at least two units of speech courses, independent of English courses, toward admission. Boards of education should be urged to adopt recommended speech texts. "Speech includes dramatics." Each of these statements reflected a worrisome problem.

ANOTHER SIGN of an expanding discipline: Textbook writers got busy.

An early college text used in the 1920s was *Effective Speaking* by Arthur Edward Phillips. Born in 1867, the author had studied classic oratory, rhetoric, and drama, in the original Latin and Greek, and from that study had deduced the principles that featured his book. "Used by over 200," the publisher's ad stated. Occasionally I borrowed a category or an example from it, so the publisher can change his figure to "over 201." Phillips' text helped bridge the transition from elocution to speech. Charles H. Woolbert's *Fundamentals of Speech* appeared in 1922; "145 institutions used it that year." One of them was Grinnell College; I studied Woolbert's text its first year as a student of John P. Ryan. When it was revised in 1927, the publisher claimed more than 1,500 adoptions. *Public Speaking* by James A. Winans, drawing from the psychology of William James and urging "conversational quality" in speech making, was widely used. W. P. Sandford and W. Hayes Yeager introduced *Principles of Effective Speaking* in 1928; its publisher brought out "three editions in less than two years." The same authors also wrote *Business and Professional Speaking*, to meet the growing demand for a text for courses with that or similar titles. In 1936 Lew Sarett and William P. Foster's *Basic Principles of Speech* and Alan H. Monroe's *Principles and Types of Speech* were published. Both were runaway best sellers. Monroe's book, with co-authors, was still a leader as the 1990's opened.

The rapidly growing number of high school speech students needed an approach suited to young speakers. Woolbert and Andrew H. Weaver's *Better Speech* came out in 1922. "This is a basic text in speech training and not one to tag along after the English work," the publishers announced, somewhat defiantly. "513 schools have adopted it—the most recent order was for 6,800 copies from Pittsburgh." 406 pages, $1.40. Alice Craig's *The Speech Arts* had a good run. Wilhemina Hedde and W. Norwood Brigance's *Speech* appeared in 1936. High schools adopted it right off, said the publisher, and it proved to be a winner.

Katharine Anne Ommanney's *The Stage and the School* was popular with high school students and teachers of drama. My copy is the third edition. Alexander M. Drummond's *A Manual of Play Production* went through at least four printings. Drummond was a fine teacher from Cornell, a big, massive, bear who walked with a cane, a peerless theater man, a pioneer in educational theater. In the 1970s I was giving a talk at a state convention and mentioned Drummond. Afterwards, a lovely lady, perhaps 50, came up and asked, "Did you actually know Drummond?" and when I said that I actually did, she gave me a tremendous hug and told me he had been her favorite teacher, and had had an immense influence on her professional life. Alex would have smiled in appreciation, and also to learn that I had been given a hug that was really meant for him.

As a high school teacher, struggling with dramatics, I leaned on these and other texts, such as John Dolman Jr.'s *The Art of Play Production* and a mimeographed edition of Alexander Dean's *Fundamentals of Play Directing*. Although Dean's pioneer work was supposed to be made available only to students of drama at Yale, I managed to get a bootlegged copy; it was helpful on the sort of detail that a beginner could snatch and put into practice.

PARALLEL WITH the formation of state associations and the writing of textbooks, for beginning and advanced courses, was the move on campuses to achieve greater recognition for the discipline.

The first two Departments of Speech to offer courses toward the Ph.D. were the University of Iowa and the University of Wisconsin, both in 1921, seven years after the national association had been founded. In his 1927 inaugural address, Association President Andrew T. Weaver, University of Wisconsin, said: "When this Association was founded 13 years ago, I doubt whether there were four similar institutions where a student could secure a bachelor's degree in speech."

In 1935, Franklin H. Knower, then of the University of Minnesota, compiled a list of graduate theses and dissertations from 1902 to 1934. The list shows the first Ph.D. was awarded in 1922; then no more until 1926, when there were 3; then 17 (later revised upwards to 19) during the five-year period 1927-1931. By the end of 1934 the total was 46. In the next 20 years—1934-1954—the total number of master's degrees awarded had increased from 642 to 6,446, and the number of doctor's degrees from 43 to 1,237. At some time during 1954, perhaps during the torrid heat of that record-breaking summer, the 1,000th Ph.D. was hooded. By 1968, the last year for which Knower compiled his annual report, 29,196 master's and 4,309 doctor's degrees had been awarded by 206 institutions; 51 had awarded doctor's degrees, including 343 new doctorates that last year.[3]

Knower ended his compilation in 1968 because it had become so massive. Year by year one can trace the progress of graduate study and learn the names of degree winners and the schools at which they studied. The annual report included the titles of masters' theses, if one had been required, and of doctors' dissertations. "Over 20,000 titles have been indexed," he wrote, probably wearily, in his final report.

NEWS ITEMS over the years showed slow but steady growth in various directions.

In the boom year of 1929, at the New York City convention, the National Association of Teachers of Speech could announce that it had distributed 3,000 copies of the first issue of *The Service Bulletin for Teachers of Speech*, primarily designed to aid teachers in the public schools. Its members listened to an extensive report of specific ways to improve the Association, with special attention to secondary schools. That year Pasadena Junior College altered its 11th year English from straight English to 3 days literature and 2 days speech education "work." ("Work" appears repeatedly; many would prefer "speech study" or "graduate study" to "speech work" or "graduate work.") A Los Angeles newspaper carried the story that the School of Speech at the University of California "is now composed of 10 faculty members, more than 1,000 students in undergraduate courses, and thirty-odd [watch that hyphen, folks] graduate students."

In February 1933 the Association heard a full report from the Committee for the Advancement of Speech Education in Elementary Schools. The University of Illinois announced that it would accept speech credits as satisfactory for entrance requirements, "thus bringing to a close the movement started by the Illinois Speech Conference at Peoria in 1930." In 1934 Louisiana high schools could offer one full unit of speech for graduation.

In 1936 the Southern Association of Teachers of Speech appointed a committee "for the purpose of trying to persuade colleges and universities to grant entrance credit for high school speech courses." In 1937 Washington University authorized the granting of a M.A. degree in English with emphasis in speech.

In 1940, Indiana University hosted the first ever National High School Drama Conference and Play Production Festival, modeled after the Interlochen Music Festival. That spring, "Masque and Gavel" was organized at Northwestern University by the faculty of the School of Speech, to recognize speech and drama activities in high schools. The University of Missouri announced a Department of Speech and Dramatic Art. Kent State University opened a School of Speech and installed a new radio workshop. And the National Association of Teachers of Speech announced its first *Directory*—well, not quite; there had been a pamphlet-type directory in 1926 that sold for a quarter.

These two ads appeared in *The Quarterly Journal of Speech Education*, June 1922, a time when most second-generation teachers of speech were high school students or college undergraduates. The Wisconsin ad gives a good idea of the courses offered by first-generation teachers of speech. Few teachers, beginners or not, will miss the realistic note in the NATS ad: "...Fee of $3.50 to be paid when salaries start next Fall."

Ads like these, showing various choices open to students, appeared in the 1920s. The same ad was frequently repeated in the early years of *The Quarterly Journal of Speech Education* (e.g., November 1923).[2]

Before long one could read about endowed chairs in the field of speech. Guggenheim awards going to speech teachers. Grants being given for research. Speech teachers becoming administrators at colleges and universities, or at schools operated by corporations (i.e. General Motors).

Finally, one began to see the profession going international. International debate had been commonplace even in the 1920s, spurred by annual visits to this country by Oxford and Cambridge teams. The Speech Communication Association welcomed members from Australia to South Africa. Its members who were directors of debate took teams overseas—Great Britain, Germany, the U.S.S.R. Others read papers at international conferences in rhetoric or education, and lectured on British, European, and Asian campuses. The International Society for the History of Rhetoric and the International Communication Association held overseas conferences with participants speaking in appropriate languages. The World Communication Association was regularly holding biennial conferences, alternating between Atlantic and Pacific sites: its 9th (1987) in Great Britain, its 10th (1989) in Singapore. Communication problems growing out of the 1989-1990 upheavals in East Germany and the rest of Eastern Europe attracted the attention of members of all of these groups.

THE COST OF PROFESSIONAL ACTIVITIES followed a monetary system that we can no longer identify with. I have a copy of a 1943 IRS return with these expenses claimed as tax-exempt:

Dues to professional associations: National Assn. of Teachers of Speech, $10.00; American Speech Correction Association, $3.00; American Association University Professors, $4.00;

Faculty club, $3.00; Eastern Public Speaking Conference, $2.00; New York State Speech Association, $1.00; total, $25.00.

Expenses of attending professional convention in New York City, $49.75

Expenses of supervising practice teachers in public schools, driving 300 miles at 5cents/mile, $15.00

The $49.75 figure included a three-day stay at The Commodore, and approximately $20.00 for a round trip ticket from Syracuse to New York City on the New York Central.

During postwar years, graduate students in the Midwest had an even better plan: to attend a Chicago convention they took capacious box lunches, prepared by their wives; the young husbands drove in one car and instead of at lodging at The Stevens, $3.50 and up, they camped out at the nearby YMCA, $1.00 a night. I would not be overly amazed if there were four or five to a room, but I have no hard evidence to present.

On a few occasions the executive secretary secured special railroad rates. For the 1934 convention in New Orleans, the Illinois Central advertised rates on the famed Panama Limited, air-conditioned throughout, leaving Chicago at 1:00 p.m., arriving in New Orleans at 9:00 a.m. One proposal covered all expenses, $69.95. At the Roosevelt Hotel rooms with bath were $3.00 and up. Now the Executive Director routinely arranges special air fares.

SO IN THESE PRE-WORLD WAR II years, the field of speech had grown in width and depth.

The national association's first convention in Chicago in 1914 drew 60 people. The

TABLE I

INSTITUTIONAL SOURCES OF DEGREES GRANTED
(1940 Degrees in Parentheses)

	MASTERS' DEGREES			DOCTORS' DEGREES		COMBINED TOTAL
	With Thesis	Without Thesis	Total			
Akron	2		2			2
Alabama	(2) 6	(1) 1	7			7
Brooklyn	14		14			14
Carnegie	11		11			11
Columbia—T. C.	3	(50) 659	662	(3)	21	683
Cornell	(15) 105		105	(3)	24	129
Denver	(8) 38		38			38
George Washington	2		2			2
Grinnel	1		1			1
Hawaii	(2) 2		2			2
Illinois	(1) 5		5			5
Indiana	(3) 5		5			5
Iowa	(50) 415		415	(3)	48	463
Louisiana	(10) 61		61	(2)	12	73
Marquette	(3) 23		23			23
Michigan	(9) 9	(39) 439	448	(5)	22	470
Minnesota	(2) 41	(1) 5	46	(1)	1	47
Missouri	(3) 6		6			6
New Mexico Normal	8		8			8
Northwestern	(5) 244	(42) 104	348	(3)	7	355
Ohio State	(7) 33		33		2	35
Ohio University	(2) 6		6			6
Ohio Wesleyan	26		26			26
Oklahoma	(3) 3		3			3
Purdue	5		5			5
South Dakota	(1) 3		3			3
Southern California	(4) 150	(38) 225	375	(6)	12	387
Stanford	21		21		1	22
Syracuse	(3) 8		8		1	9
Utah	(2) 17		17			17
Washington, University of	(4) 20		20			20
Wayne	(7) 29	(3) 9	38			38
Western Reserve	1	(11) 65	66			66
Wisconsin	(29) 242		242	(5)	42	284
Yale	(15) 42	76	118	(1)	5	123
Grand Totals	(190) 1,607	(185) 1,583	3,190	(32)	198	3,388

Franklin H. Knower published the first installment of *Index of Graduate Work in the Field of Speech* in *Speech Monographs* (1935). That installment covered the years 1902-1934. The *Index* included names of recipients and titles of theses ("thesis" included both master's thesis and doctor's dissertation). Not every department head responded to this request for information, but made sure their institutions were represented in 1936 and later issues. Titles from theater and speech pathology were included. Table I comes from *Speech Monographs* (1941).

Chicago convention of 1928 drew 354 people; it never again fell below that number. 378 came to Los Angeles in 1934. New York City drew 935 in 1937. Chicago 1,001 in 1939. Detroit 699 in 1941, the year of Pearl Harbor. After 1968, never less than 2,000 and up to 3,307, in New Orleans.

Annual membership started with 160 in 1915; 3,031 in 1935; 6,297 in 1955; 5,790 in 1975 (est.); 5,949 in 1985. The specialized associations, as in theater and speech pathology-audiology, met for a few years with the parent National Association of Teachers of Speech, and then met separately. They siphoned other thousands from the general pool once known as "speech." Even so, annual income reached $136,824 in 1963, the last year the Association was quartered on a university campus and managed by a university-based executive secretary.[4] In 1963 the Association appointed a full time executive secretary, moved its office from the campus of Indiana University to New York City, and then eventually to Annandale, Virginia, entering the 1990s with an income in seven figures. The title of the official in charge was changed

TABLE II

NUMBER OF DEGREES GRANTED WITH AND WITHOUT THESIS TABULATED BY YEAR

YEAR	MASTERS' DEGREES				DOCTORS' DEGREES	
	With Thesis	Without Thesis	Total	Percent of Total	Number	Percent
1902	1		1	.03134		
1903	1		1	.03134		
1904	1		1	.03134		
1906	1		1	.03134		
1907	1		1	.03134		
1908	3		3	.09404		
1909	1		1	.03134		
1912	1		1	.03134		
1913	1		1	.03134		
1917	1		1	.03134		
1918	1	1	2	.06269		
1920	3	1	4	.12539		
1921	2		2	.06269		
1922	7	1	8	.25078	1	.50505
1923	9	3	12	.37617		
1924	19	6	25	.78369		
1925	28	16	44	1.37931		
1926	37	18	55	1.72413	3	1.51515
1927	43	19	62	1.94357	1	.50505
1928	38	25	63	1.97492	5	2.52525
1929	88	40	128	4.01253	4	2.02020
1930	79	66	145	4.54545	6	3.03030
1931	113	53	166	5.20376	2	1.01010
1932	96	101	197	6.17554	11	5.55555
1933	84	128	212	6.64576	8	4.04040
1934	78	153	231	7.24137	7	3.53535
1935	104	113	217	6.80250	14	7.07070
1936	122	142	264	8.27586	21	10.60606
1937	131	170	301	9.43573	28	14.14141
1938	172	171	343	10.75235	28	14.14141
1939	151	171	322	10.09404	27	13.63636
1940	190	185	375	11.75548	32	16.16161
Totals	1,607	1,583	3,190	99.99982	198	99.99995

By 1932, the year of Roosevelt's first election, 33 doctor's degrees had been awarded. By 1934 there were 48, one for each state. By 1940, the year of the third-term election, 165. The requirement to demonstrate a "reading knowledge" of French and German for the doctorate was almost inescapable. Another language could be substituted but only for a demonstrable reason. Later, statistics could be substituted. Gradually other changes were made. Table II comes from *Speech Monographs* (1941).

to Executive Director. Andy Weaver, who gave the 1927 presidential address cited above, to an audience of perhaps 150, would have been astounded. And Cornell's "Chief" Winans, of the original 17 founders, who liked to tell about walking down Michigan Boulevard with the total assets of the National Association of Academic Teachers of Public Speaking in his coat pocket, would have called it nothing less than a miracle.

LATE IN 1940 a statement appeared in *The Quarterly Journal of Speech* that describes at least in part the motivation for the activities I have narrated:

The tremendous importance of speech education grows on the imagination of the general public year by year. But when it becomes more generally understood that practically every bit of progress the human race has made—the publishing of every good book, the establishment of every great library, the building of every school, the creation of every factory, the laying of every highway, and the erection of every church—has been brought about by the earnest plea of some fine man or woman, or of some group of men and women, using the persuasion of speech, then speech education will achieve its proper recognition. It is of high value not only for its own merits but because it stimulates every other form of education and broadens every student who delves into it with the purpose of self-improvement.[5]

The author was Arthur J. Wiltse, manager of the Ann Arbor Press, printer and publisher of "books, magazines, and general printing," and of *The Quarterly Journal of Speech*. I never met Mr. Wiltse, but we must have known scores of the same people.

ALTHOUGH MY TEACHING was in speech, I was still a member of a Department of English. This situation bothered me partly because the title of "Assistant Professor of English" did not describe what I was doing. Moreover, the academic ventures we proposed needed such careful explaining and justification within the Department before we could take them to higher levels. Getting funds to buy new apparatus (professors of Chaucer and Milton never needed apparatus) or to get approval for a new course (which would be ex-pan-sion) met formidable obstacles.

About that time Syracuse University, one of the few institutions that had a School of Speech, wrote me about an opening. I saw a chance to have a title not merely in a Department of Speech but in a School of Speech. I could abandon speech pathology and debating and concentrate on rhetoric and public address. The lure of being more of a specialist had got to me; I could be less of a one-man band. The Syracuse catalog showed an array of courses far beyond our expectations at Missouri. It even had courses in radio broadcasting, taught in a campus studio with access to the facilities of a commercial station. It had a theater program with close ties to Broadway. A student could take a master's degree without taking courses in English unless he wished.

I did not want to leave the university of my native state if the doors that seemed so tightly closed could be jarred loose, but got little encouragement when I visited with the head of the Department of English. We walked down the hall to the office of the dean of the college and these two patriarchs, department head and dean, both close to retirement, conferred in private while I roosted outside, wondering why I was not invited to argue my own future. Before long the department head emerged with the message that I was welcome to stay, but that Missouri would compete just so much.

To make the move, Gus and I traded for a shiny, new, black Chevrolet sedan. In September, with our wee ones—now two in number—we began the drive across the country.

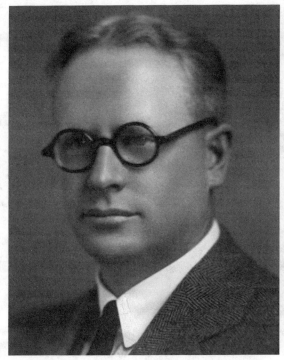

James M. O'Neil, SCA President 1915

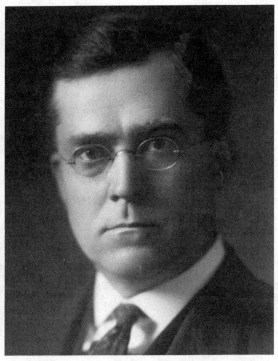

James A. Winans, SCA President 1916

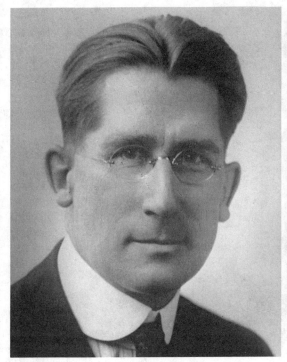

Charles. H. Woolbert, SCA President 1920

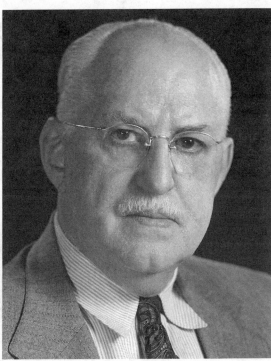

A. M. Drummond, SCA President 1921

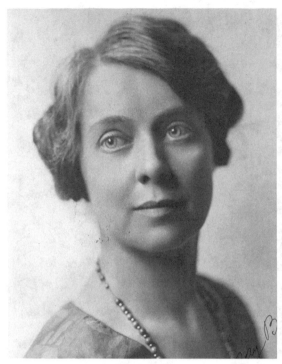

Maud May Babcock, SCA President 1936

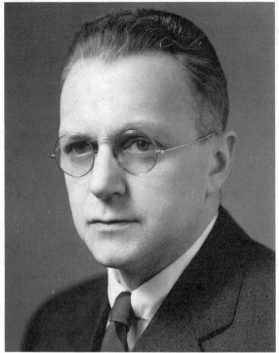

Herbert A. Wichelns, SCA President 1937

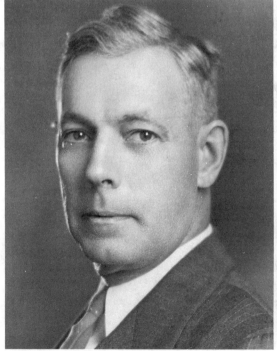

A. Craig Baird, SCA President 1939

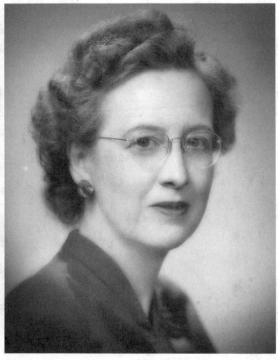

Magdalene Kramer, SCA President 1947

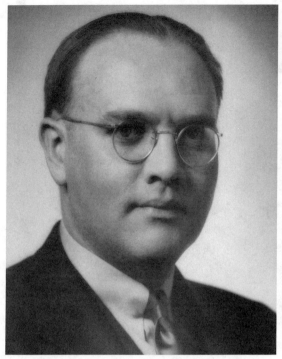

Wilbur Gilman, SCA President 1951

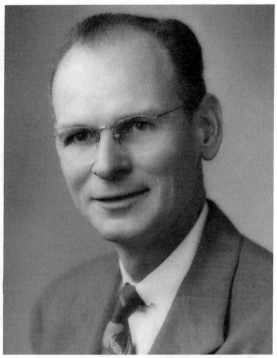

Lester Thonssen, SCA President 1956

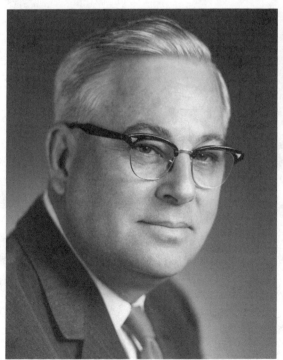

Waldo W. Braden, SCA President 1962

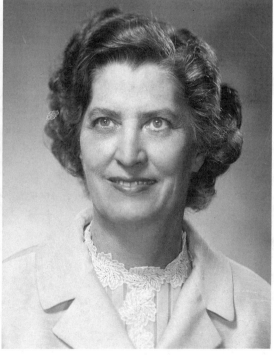

Marie Hochmuth Nichols, SCA President 1969

Teaching Speech: Wartime

NOW WE WERE UNDERTAKING our longest journey, most of the way following aging Highway 40, through Illinois, Indiana, Ohio, town by town, one Main Street after another. In each town we heard radios booming the bulletins about the war in Europe. On September 1, a few days before we had begun our trip, Hitler had started his blitz across the face of Poland; two days later Britain and France had declared war. Hitler's panzer divisions seemed to travel as fast as we did. By the time we entered New York, Poland's doom was certain. Western civilization braced itself for World War II. We braced ourselves for our new job, not in a Department of English but in a School of Speech. We were looking forward to a new phase of our lives, but segments of our minds wondered what the conflict overseas would mean to our own country.

LOCATED IN A CITY of 205,000, Syracuse University enrolled 4,800 students and had a faculty half again the size we had left. Its meager budget had barely survived the stresses of the Great Depression but it was now rebuilding its faculty, with fifteen new appointments. The School of Speech was then one of the thirty-five places in the country offering graduate degrees; it had averaged three M.A.'s a year. It was located on the third floor of the Hall of Languages, one of the oldest buildings on campus. (Young disciplines are often housed in aged structures on top floors or in basements.) It had its own library, also on the third floor. Its strongest areas were radio, theater, and public speaking; it would soon have an impressive area in speech pathology. Its weakest, oral interpretation, was still rooted in the Age of Elocution.

I introduced a course in rhetorical criticism and later received a dual appointment with the School of Education to teach speech education and to supervise practice teaching. In this area I could draw upon high school experience; most professors of speech education had never actually taught in the public schools.

I also had two classes in public speaking, one of them for students in the College of Engineering, which had decided only recently that its students would now be required to add this course. This sudden change in the rules created a hubbub. As I was in my office, awaiting the students on the first day, I heard male voices and a heavy rumble of feet stomping up the stairway.

—Where's this goddam public speaking class? Grumble, grumble.

—Who's the goddam prof, anyway? Mutter, mutter. Variety of mixed responses, not entirely clear— probably fortunately.

Obvious, extra loud tramping into the room, and heavy rearrangement of chairs.

I waited a moment and entered the room, facing 2 1/2 dozen of the mutineers.

I looked over the group, all male. "I have an office just across the hall," I said, "and as I was waiting, I heard voices saying, I'm not exactly sure what, but something like, 'Where's this goddam public speaking class?'" Over the room I began to see bits and pieces of grins. "And then I heard some voices saying, 'Who's the goddam prof?'

"I think those are gentlemanly questions, gentlemanly stated, and I'll try to answer them."

I wrote my name on the board, commented that it was often misspelled, made brief identifying statements, and then talked about public speaking. An engineer, a member of one of the oldest professions, is often called upon to explain his ideas to other professionals, sometimes in technical, sometimes in non-technical language; but to laymen, in non-technical language. He owes it to himself to be able to speak as clearly and meaningfully as he can. What he says may result in his getting, or not getting, a contract. In life there is often no second prize—they choose you, or they choose the other person. You are not about to be taught anything fancy or eloquent, but you will be given a chance to be as interesting and as persuasive as you can be.

Since you have already demonstrated that you are a lively, animated group, you will probably do better at speechmaking than you expect.

We had a good time together. At the end of the semester the class had a picnic, inviting their dates and Gus and me. Fifty years have come and gone and I have forgotten every name, every face, but the group impression persists. War came the next year and called them off the campus. I have wondered if their improved communicative skills served them well in their military or non-military situations, and afterwards in civic and professional situations.

SYRACUSE MEMORIES are an inseparable mix of personal events and the war in Europe. We had already planned to add to our family, and waited apprehensively through the "phony war" that followed the invasion of Poland. Then, in May, 1940, tanks and Stuka dive bombers roared through the Low Countries. About the time Gus entered the hospital, the Germans unexpectedly outflanked the vaunted Maginot Line, and had France reeling. Troops entered Paris on June 15; Americans were numbed and bewildered.

That same June 15, Stephen Reid entered the University Hospital. I took a copy of the morning newspaper with its unbelievable headlines, PARIS SURRENDERS, to Gus's room. We were so shaken that for a moment we almost forgot the new boy. And when we did remember him, we said, simply, "What a time to bring a baby into the world." Before Gus went home, after the usual ten-day stay, the heart of France had been struck from the free world.

The battles were so gigantic they were named, not after hills or groves or towns, but after countries. The Battle of France was followed by the sky war to be known as the Battle of Britain. Trying desperately to defend against the waves of bombers, British troops were shooting out the linings of their anti-aircraft guns. I was with a group of professors who were certain that Britain would fall. A Canadian among us insisted: "Britain will not fall. The British are tough. They'll hang on." He brushed our doubts aside. "I'm Canadian. I know them better than you do." Of course he was right. Years later, in England on a raw, wet day, we heard an American voice: "I don't know why Hitler ever thought he could lick the British when they've been through centuries of this kind of weather."

What we did not fully realize then was that with the new developments in radar the Royal Air Force could operate at the peak of efficiency. And years later, reading history from the viewpoint of a teacher, I could not help noting that in the early part of the war the Nazis had poured not only their pilots but the instructors of the pilots into the conflict, losing many, and thus so weakening their training program that new crops of pilots got only half as much training and were far less capable than their British or American counterparts.

My student speakers argued that America should stay neutral. "This is a European conflict," they declared. "We got dragged in once before; when we left, the situation got worse than ever; this time we must keep out."

Politics heated up and Roosevelt was renominated; the Republicans selected Wendell Willkie. At issue was the third term. As most states went Democratic, leaving only New York and a few others for the Republicans, the result was a landslide.

Congress debated whether or not to renew the draft; my students became avid readers of newspapers. So heated was the debate that the House of Representatives passed the act by a single vote, the first peacetime draft in our history. Because this war was using more machinery—aircraft, tanks, radio sets—than other wars, the decision was made early to apply the principle of "selective" service: people were as necessary to build the war machine as to operate it in the field; our troops and those of our allies needed to be both fed and clothed. When war actually came, we were poorly prepared as it was; the lead time afforded by that 1940 act was one of those serendipitous miracles of history.

The day came when millions of men up to age 35 were called upon to register. I appeared before our local board and received a card to carry in my wallet—in fact I bought a wallet in order to have something to carry the card in. Since I was married, had three children, and was doing useful work. I received a deferred rating because, as the phrase read, "of fatherhood and other hardships."

THAT FALL I had my first opportunity to contribute to a convention of the National Association of Teachers of Speech. A. Craig Baird had been elected president, and in connection with the meeting in Chicago, he asked me to be in charge of "banquets, luncheons, and public relations." That invitation was not so handsome as being invited to give the keynote address, but I was as pleased as if it had been. I wrote the chef at The Stevens reminding him that an important event on his December calendar was to prepare a convention banquet for us, and asking him to send sample menus. He responded promptly with a list of offerings. I passed up the heavy stuff he was featuring that season for $7.50, thought we could do better than the minimum $2.50 offering, and wrote him that we would take the chicken Kiev for $2.75. I did not know precisely what chicken Kiev was, but it sounded warlike, or at least European. His reply indicated his pleasure with my choice, and asked me kindly to indicate how many settings I would guarantee. His letter had a bit of a grim note since if, for example, I guaranteed more customers than I delivered, the Association, or me, I wasn't sure which, would have to fork up the shortage. Even worse, if I guaranteed too few, and starving members had to be turned away, the finger of shame would be pointed at you-know-who. He did, however, offer a leeway of 10 tickets in either direction.

I reflected that previous Chicago conventions had drawn from 500 to 900 registrants. Trying to visualize the usual banquet attendance, I decided that a third of those registered might attend the luncheon. I wrote the chef that I would guarantee 300 tickets.

Afterwards, the more I reflected, the more positive I was that we would not sell nearly that many. To help salvage a desperate outlook, I sent a letter to a long list of probable convention attenders, describing as enticingly as I could the meal that The Stevens' chef was preparing, and other features of the banquet.

You can imagine that when I arrived in Chicago I kept showing up at the ticket desk to count the prospects. The evening before the banquet we were 100 tickets short. I could be liable for as much as $275. Next morning sales were slow, but just before the zero hour business picked up. With 1,001 present, the attendance at the convention was the largest in the history of the Association. And as 295 of them showed up at the luncheon, both the chef and I were pleased.

Ever since, when I have attended any banquet, large or small, public or private, I have quietly said to myself, "Some poor devil has had to guarantee a figure, and is hoping the attendance will come within the plus-or-minus-10 safety net." I suspect that poor devil has a title, like Executive Director, or it may be a close friend, your host or hostess.

IN THE SUMMER OF 1941 people had talked seriously about the probability of our involvement in the war, which would speed up the draft and bring shortages and disruptions. Families did more canning than usual. Many still remembered World War I, with rationing of sugar and flour and scarcity of other commodities. Once again the country might face quotas and coupons. Gus canned a hundred quarts of tomatoes, along with green beans, peaches, plums, pears—anything she could locate in groceries or orchards.

Older men, even those with families, found themselves being re-classified and thus becoming more likely to be called up. The military was dipping deeper and deeper into its manpower pool, summoning to active duty men who had thus far been deferred. I was elevated from 3B to 3A—"until further notice."

On a December Sunday afternoon, like millions of others, we were tuned to newscaster Lowell Thomas. Pearl Harbor had been attacked. We were stunned. As the hours went by the news grew steadily worse. Before we went to bed, we knew we had suffered a military disaster. The European situation was alarming enough; Pearl Harbor made the disaster global.

A single hostile act of Japan had galvanized us into war.

Monday, December 8, I met my early morning class in public speaking. Not a single student was absent. The assignment had been to make entertaining speeches, but nobody felt like being entertaining. No one expected that we would have much of a class, but all felt the urge to carry on, doing what they had been doing, until they knew something better to do. For a while we sat and looked at each other; then we began to share what few news bulletins we had heard; we told each other where we had been when we heard about the disaster. The next class, in rhetorical theory, talked not about Aristotle's *Rhetoric* but about Pearl Harbor.

At noon the President addressed Congress.

"Yesterday, December 7, 1941—a date which will live in infamy—the United States of America was suddenly and deliberately attacked by naval and air forces of Japan." And so on to: "With confidence in our armed forces—with the unbounded determination of our people—we will gain the inevitable triumph— so help us God."

Over the radio—TV was yet to come—we could hear the mighty ovation that followed, the shouts of "Vote, vote!" and later the result: 82-0 in the Senate, 388-1 in the House. Within four hours the resolution had been passed and signed.[1]

The largest audience ever to hear a radio program listened to the American president in this masterpiece of communication and leadership. Around the world, people tuned in. Repeatedly we heard the phrase, "total mobilization."

By Wednesday the campus had pulled itself together. The underlying mood had completely altered; I heard no more talk about staying out of the war. A student named Barney told me he was going to enlist in the Coast Guard. "The next meeting will be my last class," he said. I knew students would begin to leave and I was deeply moved. "Barney, we'll end the next hour with a farewell speech from you." This comment shows a teacher at work, trying to devise a real-life assignment. Barney left with our good wishes, our hopes, and all sorts of personal messages.

Barney was the first of many. After Christmas, enrollment diminished rapidly. A class of twenty would dwindle to fifteen, then ten. Many campuses gave full credit, whether or not the semester were actually completed. Some students enlisted; some went into war work. An expeditionary army would need not only people but all kinds of gear: clothing, ammunition, food. Girls dropped out as well as fellows. We heard a succession of farewell speeches; each one was an expression of what it was like to tear away from family, friends, school. "Keep Syracuse as it is until I come back," was a common theme.

We pledged that we would, but how could we? Already we had lived through a social and technological revolution, but that was just a starter to what lay ahead: disruption, dislocation, and destruction on a scale that would destroy millions and alter forever the lives of those who survived.

IT WAS AN EXCITING TIME to teach communication when so much exciting, world-wide talk was going on. I have mentioned Roosevelt; the world was more and more becoming aware of the genius of Winston Churchill. Candor is among the higher virtues of communication, whether the situation is public or private, and he never pulled his punches. In his first year as prime minister he had made one eloquent address after another. "I have nothing to offer but blood, tears, toil, and sweat," he had warned, on taking office. After the Dunkirk disaster he had thundered: "We shall fight on the seas and oceans, . . . we shall fight on the beaches, we shall fight on the landing grounds, we shall fight in the fields and in the streets, we shall fight in the hills, we shall never surrender." Here was gleaming, shining courage, uttered when western Europe was falling apart. (During the applause that followed he is reported to have muttered, "And we will fight the sons of bitches with beer bottles, which is all we have got.")

In the spring of 1941 I had been invited to read a paper at the upcoming December speech convention at Detroit—"talk on any aspect of British rhetoric you wish," the letter had said. I replied that I would discuss Churchill as a speaker.

In preparation I read everything available about Churchill's early speaking career. I studied his appearances in the newsreels. I wrote British statesmen who might supply information. I needed details that would explain how he developed his art of speaking, a kind of information not easy to come by.

I was intrigued to discover that his desire to master English went back as far as his prep school days. As he had seemed totally unable to comprehend Latin, his masters had made him take a double dose of English. Failure to know Latin kept him out of Cambridge or Oxford but he qualified for a military school, and thus got an education of sorts. When he was stationed in India, he read widely in ethics, philosophy, and literature—-partly so he could converse intelligently with other officers, most of whom were Oxford or Cambridge men, but mainly because he developed a considerable appetite for reading. When he entered the House of Commons, he rehearsed his speeches diligently. As he realized he was not effective in spur-of-the-moment rebuttal, he prepared three or four speeches for each debate, hoping that one of them would fit the arguments of the opposition. In short, few people have worked harder to master the art of speaking well. An ancient comment is that orators are born, not made. Churchill's experience and that of countless others shows that natural gifts are just dandy but plain old toil is what gets the job done.

At the time of Pearl Harbor, Churchill's brilliance as a speaker was not well known to the American public. A week before the Detroit convention, Churchill came to the United States and addressed a joint session of Congress. The speech was magnificent. At the last minute I had been able to secure a segment of news film showing Churchill in action.

Among those present at the convention session were Detroit area reporters. The man from Associated Press picked up a tiny excerpt from my talk that Churchill's having failed Latin was a reason for his having become proficient in speechmaking. Since he had been required to take extra courses in English, he thus, as he himself put it, had got a firm grasp on the magic and power of the English sentence. The rest of my argument was overlooked, but this quote from the AP dispatch was printed nation-wide. The *Des Moines Register* put a seven-column headline over a six-inch story about this fine British speaker who had failed Latin. As Churchill might have said, never in the field of human communication was so large a headline erected over so small a story.

WHEN WILBUR GILMAN was called up as a first lieutenant in the Coast Artillery in 1942, he resigned his position as book review editor of the *Quarterly Journal of Speech*, and the editor, W. Norwood Brigance, asked me to take the post. In his job description of the responsibilities of a book review editor he wrote that it "requires an unsuspected amount of labor, patience, and skill." The holder must keep in touch with "scores of publishers," "select qualified and able reviewers," "and—here's the rub—persuade them to write a review by a certain time and of a certain length." Above all, whatever happens, come what may, he must deliver copy to the editor on the deadline date.[2]

I edited the department for a couple of years and more or less did the bulk of the above. Being on the lookout for good titles in drama and speech pathology, as well as in public speaking and rhetoric, and having only eight pages available, I limited reviews to 800 words, in order to get the pick of the lot. At times reviewers complained, and at times I grudgingly yielded an extra 200 words or so. Over the years when I have read a review that was unbearably long, on a book of mild significance or on a subject that would attract few readers, I have thought the policy of brief reviews to be good.

THE 1943 CONVENTION of the National Association of Teachers of Speech was billed as a War Problems Conference. A general session and several sectional meetings were planned to consider topics like: War and Post-War Problems of NATS. Radio, Education, and the War. The Theater in War-Time. Speech Instruction for Members of the Armed Forces.The conference was held in New York, at The Commodore, a big barn of a hotel that was popular with academic groups. Because of the movement of members of the armed forces and their families, travel by rail was so congested that the government had asked associations to limit or shorten their meetings. A copy of the 30-page, pocket-size, convention program still exists in the Association's national office. The "Call to Conference" is couched in solemn language:

> Even a casual glance at the program for The National Association of Teachers of Speech
> will show that the meeting is devoted primarily to the war effort. . . . In undertaking to schedule

a conference this year, the executives of The National Association of Teachers of Speech have carefully refrained from promoting a large and casual attendance at the meeting. . . .

Anyone who attends the War Problems Conference is on public business and should attend strictly to that business. . . . Meetings must and will begin and close on schedule. Those who plan to attend the meetings should be in their seats promptly at the hour set. . . . Members should not plan to leave New York City before the close of the last meeting on Thursday, December 30, at 6:00 p.m.

An event held in connection with the convention luncheon was the formal presentation to the Association of the two volumes of the *History and Criticism of American Public Address*, which brought together research on the leading speakers of three centuries, each chapter written by a teacher of speech who had specialized on a selected speaker, and edited by Brigance. Included were five articles on historical background and 29 articles on outstanding speakers from Jonathan Edwards to Woodrow Wilson. The volumes were presented by Curtis Benjamin, president of McGraw-Hill Publishing Co., and accepted by Joseph F. Smith of the University of Utah.

I was billed as the luncheon speaker, and commented on the problem of getting accurate reports of speeches, with special mention of the problem of wartime policy speeches, wartime state papers, and wartime communique's. I drew upon experiences as member of a newspaper family that covered local speeches, and as Linotype operator in the Government Printing Office, setting speeches that had been delivered in Congress but afterwards had been heavily edited by the senator or representative before being printed in the *Congressional Record*. I could see on the sheets themselves that the speaker, and later a Government Printing Office editor, had not only corrected grammar and sentence structure, but had also revised or rearranged whole sections.[3]

The Brigance volumes honored that day were the first of many books sponsored by the Association, in which selected contributors pooled their research by writing articles on a central theme. Despite the cost—$10.00 for the two-volume set—2,000 sets were sold by 1956, with second-hand sets going for $35 to $50. A third volume on great American speakers was issued, edited by Marie Hochmuth of the University of Illinois, and published by Longmans, Green and Company. She presented the volumes to the Association at the 1955 Los Angeles convention, and they were accepted in behalf of the Association by Waldo W. Braden, executive secretary.[4]

Later, other volumes were published that dealt with speakers or issues of national or regional importance. One ambitious undertaking was *History of Speech Education in America*, edited by Karl R. Wallace, with 36 contributors writing a background section, a section on rhetoric, elocution, and speech, and a section on educational theater. In the decades that followed were numerous other titles, including several written in honor of distinguished professors (e.g. Winans, Baird, Wichelns, Wise).[5]

IN THOSE DECADES, the most distinguished Department of Speech in the East was at Cornell University. At conventions I had met such luminaries as Herbert A. Wichelns and Russell Wagner (rhetoric), Alexander M. Drummond (theater), and C. K. Thomas (phonetics), so I made a special trip to Ithaca to renew the acquaintance. At a luncheon at which teachers from Ithaca College and the local schools were also invited, a passing reference was made to the fact that the Empire State did not yet have a speech association. Licensing of speech teachers still had to cross the desk of the supervisor for English in the state department of education, who insisted that anyone who had had courses in literature, plus a little gumption, could teach speech and direct debates and plays.

I mentioned that the Missouri association had confronted problems like these, and the group decided the time had come to organize a New York state speech association. The messenger who brings bad news is executed, but the messenger bearing good news is given a job. Came a day when, in a smoke-filled room, I was nominated to be president of the new association.

We knew the new New York State Speech Association could do little while the war was on, but we could make a start. Despite declining enrollments and depleted numbers of teachers, we had a state-wide conference in 1942 at the Hall of Languages on the Syracuse campus. I recall the dimly lighted auditorium, the tiny group present: the secretary, Eleanor Luse of Wells College, competent and efficient, soon to move to the University of Vermont (in that period of time the secretary of an organization was invariably a woman), Wagner and others from Cornell, Mardel Ogilvie of State Teachers College, Fredonia, later of Queens College (during any discussion Mardel would be there to remind us that we must not forget elementary school teachers in our planning), Syracuse colleagues Milton Dickens and Edward McEvoy, and others from high school and college I well knew then but have forgotten over the years. We were clinging to a few shreds of our profession while adjusting ourselves to the war.

In March of 1943 we published the first issue of our *News Bulletin*. We appointed an Executive Council of 28 members, making sure that every level of instruction and every specialty, was represented. At the 1943 New York convention, the "War Problems Conference" mentioned above, we had, one evening, what we called our first official meeting. We adopted constitution and by-laws, elected officers (Reid, president; Ogilvie, vice-president; Luse, secretary), and an executive council of 21 members. We claimed a membership of 270.[6]

In March 1967, the New York State Speech Association held its 25th Anniversary Convention at the elegant Park Sheraton Hotel in New York City.

The silver anniversary president, J. Edward McEvoy, invited me to come to New York City and speak at the banquet. I was emotionally stirred when I entered the hotel, saw the crowd around the registration table, greeted familiar faces. In the large exhibition hall I saw twenty or thirty booths staffed by representatives of publishing houses, recording machine makers, suppliers of theater equipment. More people were at the head table of the banquet than were at that last meeting at which I had presided. Afterwards, McEvoy wrote me a thank-you note hoping that I would personally be able to attend the 50th anniversary meeting. I replied that I hoped that in 1992 we could again be seated at the head table. 1992—not a bad year for anniversaries, considering that it is also the 500th anniversary of the discovery of America. But now, back to 1942.

SYRACUSE UNIVERSITY'S School of Speech, which long had offered a master's degree, sought approval for the doctorate. Although only two members of the staff held the Ph.D., we did not think this shortcoming a grave disadvantage. The field had been developed by men and women who held master's degrees or less. These years the whole of New York state had only fifteen or twenty Ph.D.'s in our discipline.

We presented our case to the Graduate Council. A dozen professors had gathered to hear our proposal. To them *speech* was synonymous with *elocution*. What was this *speech*? what was its substance? what did we actually teach? A discipline has to present its case continually. Moreover, in these critical times, the Council was reluctant to expand anything. And its members, particularly Floyd H. Allport, well-known social psychologist, thought our proposal would have been stronger if we had sought approval only for quantitative studies in public speaking and group discussion; two of these Allport had helped to sponsor. We wanted, however, to pave the way also for historical and critical studies.

We showed the group a copy of *The Quarterly Journal of Speech*, which now had been published for a quarter of a century, a copy of *Speech Monographs*, and statistics about state, regional, and national associations. As a profession we were a going concern. We could report that 42 institutions had already awarded 4,200 master's degrees and 300 Ph.D.'s.

We had brought along the recently-published 800-page *Bibliography of Speech Education*, compiled by Lester Thonssen and Elizabeth Fatherson. We read a list of major areas under which its thousands of titles were indexed. "We would like to have your approval to sponsor doctorates in our whole area," we said, in effect. "We do not want to have to come back and ask for bits and pieces. For each of our candidates the graduate dean and faculty will select the supervising committee, as is done in all areas. This committee can say yes or no to each dissertation proposal, just as it does in every other field of study.

"We want to recruit outstanding graduate students nationwide, and we will not be able to do so unless we can make them feel that the climate here is favorable."

Questions were asked; the *Journal* and other materials circulated; for a while several conversations were going on at the same time. One could feel that a consensus was in the making, and the decision to give us the green light was reached almost without a formal vote.

From a large pool of candidates, the School awarded fellowships and teaching assistantships, to students who brought sparkle and enthusiasm to the underclass courses they taught. When war broke out, however, fellows and assistants left for wartime duties. Our new program was a casualty of the war, not to be revived for half a decade.

WHEREVER WE TURNED, we faced wartime conditions. With gasoline rationed, many people turned to bicycles. I visited a shop that was down to its last bicycle, a used one, and bought it for $8. I also bought the dealer's last tire.

At first I thought I would never manage the seven miles from our new home in suburban Fayetteville to the University. In those days, bikes did not have gearshifts. Astonishingly enough, however, in a week I felt more hopeful. Large muscles build rapidly and before long I was pedaling nonstop to the campus. Arriving on campus, I leaned my bicycle, unchained, unlocked, against the side of the Hall of Languages.

Folk from suburban districts could also use an ancient groaning bus, generally so full of passengers that it looked like those seen in India or Turkey, with people clinging to every conceivable hand hold. I worried freely about that bus, my alternate way home, especially at night. As a boy growing up in a small town newspaper I knew the sounds of machinery in distress. The dark blue exhaust from the bus was warning enough but the prolonged rumbling from its bowels whenever the driver shifted gears was ominous. At the end of every trip I would reflect, Well, we escaped disaster today but probably not tomorrow.

Students and others took volunteer wartime short courses: Gus took one in first aid, becoming part of the reserve pool that could be summoned in the event of disaster. At home she demonstrated the art of bandaging; the kids liked to have her put their arms in slings or swathe their heads in gauze. They also practiced on Gus. I was shaken the first time I came home and saw a whole family heavily bandaged.

The demand for machinists was so great—"Help Wanted" ads screamed messages like "Turret Lathes Will Win the War"—that I got a job at the local Precision Casting Company, working three nights a week, and spent hours standing at a drill press or a milling machine helping make high-tech aluminum parts for artillery and submarines. Most of my co-workers had had no previous experience with production-line machinery. Even so, one applicant, asked if she had had any experience with machinery, had promptly replied: "Yes, of course, sewing machine and washing machine." We all had to learn, but we got the job done, to the satisfaction of the sharp-eyed inspectors.

SO MANY STUDENTS left for war or war work that within months enrollment was down to half. Faculty members resigned. A few qualified for commissions in their specialties: historians became military historians, physical education instructors and coaches supervised fitness programs andcoached service teams, psychologists studied learning in military situations, lawyers and others went into the Judge Advocate's or the Quartermaster's branch. Along the way most of them got a heavy dose of infantry drill combined with calisthenics, and other military activity before moving to their permanent assignments.

Total war demands all kinds of expertise; many who taught physics, languages, chemistry, meteorology, engineering, mathematics, moved from the classroom either to the armed force's training program or to the nation's industry that was rapidly tooling up for war production.

An instructor in political science joined the paratroopers. He seemed too quiet, reserved, and unassuming to enlist in a hazardous military unit. When I saw him on furlough, I asked, in awe, how many times he had jumped. "Six," he said, proudly. "Notice I don't say, 'only six'; I say, 'six.'" I find myself wondering how many times he eventually jumped, and if he jumped once too often.

On the campuses, students formed Red Cross chapters, participated in mass calisthenics, took more wrestling, boxing, and commando-type courses in physical education—and less tennis, golf, and archery. Many enrolled in courses in a foreign language, including newly organized classes in Russian.

Pep rallies were transformed into War Bond drives. Student government diminished in importance or vanished altogether. More women, fewer men, were on debate teams; subjects appeared like "Women's Place in the War." Many groups suspended activities for the duration. There were fewer all-school dances and lavish parties.

College annuals printed lists of those killed in the war and reported memorial services held on the campus. Student publications felt the rising cost of newsprint, the decrease in national advertising, the difficulty of obtaining photographic materials.

The word "acceleration" appeared frequently. Traditional prerequisites disappeared. On many campuses a student could be graduated in two full years and eight months. Young men, uncertain when they would be called up, wanted to get as close to graduation as possible. Young women, just as unsure of the future, took extra courses, attended summer school.

CHANCELLOR AND DEANS called our shrinking faculty together and warned us that the University might shut down altogether or operate with a fragment of its normal staff. Then they learned that in this guns-not-butter war, certain to last years, the armed forces could use the nation's colleges and universities to train large numbers of troops. Campuses could provide dormitories, fraternity and sorority houses, eating facilities. Military officers would supply the combat training; professors would instruct in basic skills. Mathematics. English. Public speaking. Meteorology. Geography. Hygiene and first aid. These moves a nation makes when it girds itself for survival. We were not in a settlers-and-Indians war; we were training civilians to use sophisticated weapons against an enemy that had a head start.

By the scores, college and university presidents and business executives converged on Washington and cooled their heels in the anterooms of procurement officers, sitting alongside captains of industry who were also seeking contracts. Syracuse's chancellor William S. Tolley was among the first of university administrators to offer facilities to the armed forces. The Air Force sent the University 1,050 cadets in March 1943, (thirty-five "flights" of 30 students) and another 1,050 later, the University buying houses and apartment buildings near the campus to supplement the rapidly emptying fraternity houses and dormitories. At one time we heard the rumor that the University had bought 18 houses; that was only the beginning. Once Tolley got a distress call from Washington; 550 army cadets were on a train, enroute to a college campus that found it would be unable to accept them. Acting promptly, he found it possible to house them at Auburn Theological Seminary, which had closed its doors for lack of students, and which was about a half-hour drive from Syracuse. The request came on a Monday, and the cadets moved in on a Wednesday; I find myself wondering if they spent the intervening two days on the train—perhaps, for example, to Chicago and back.[7] The initiative and imagination with which the University team worked was typical of American energy and enterprise, American determination to fight the war on all fronts.

Before long, Syracuse University had 3,800 army and air force students, men and women, to look after. Faculty members, regardless of specialty, prepared to teach courses like those listed above. A professor of mathematics could move into arithmetic but a professor of medieval history might have to teach geography. Some made the shift better than others. I heard wild stories like that of the professor of corporation law who taught navigation—from his law notes. I just missed being recycled as a meteorologist but instead became an English teacher and was assigned sections in basic grammar and composition. Each section met two hours daily. All of this was in addition to regular teaching loads.

My first class in Aircrew English met at 7:00 a.m. The cadets had been roused at 6:00, had had calisthenics and breakfast; then each flight was marched to class. They filed into my classroom on the third floor of the Hall of Languages. As soon as the bell rang, I stepped inside the classroom; they rose to their feet and stood at attention. The section marcher saluted: "Squadron 3, flight 1, reporting for instruction, sir." I returned the salute and said, "Gentlemen, be seated."

We worked systematically through the Air Force manuals, which I thought were excellent, checking home work and in general trying to teach the writing of sentences and paragraphs that made sense. Cadets were attentive in class and eager to learn. After two hours, I asked the section marcher to prepare the group for dismissal. They stood, we saluted, and he marched them from the room, row by row. They were careful to break step as they descended the creaking, wooden stairway.

Cadets marched to their classes singing popular songs. They were serious about their studies and had a full schedule, including instruction in hygiene, navigation, physical culture, and drill. And of course, instruction in flying. If any one fell asleep in class we were supposed to report him, and he would be required to march three hours on Sunday morning on the parade ground. The resident college men and women were much intrigued by the presence of the cadets on the campus, and a lot of chatter went on between the two groups. One cadet, marching in line, called out to a student in civilian clothes, "Why aren't you in uniform," and he replied, "Well, I could count up to four but I couldn't sing." One day a bunch of women got together and marched to class singing "Glory, glory hallelujah." On a football Saturday the Syracuse cadets cheered for Cornell and the Cornell naval cadets cheered for Syracuse. In general the college women got along fine with both the Air Force and the Navy.

ONE DAY THE STUDENTS ASKED: "Sir, we have learned you are a teacher of public speaking. We are officer candidates and will have to do a lot of oral presentations and briefings. Could we occasionally have suggestions about doing this?"

As their proposal made good sense, I was happy to agree. Along with talk about the agreement of subject and predicate, I could help with the selection and organization of ideas and their oral presentation.

After the course was completed, I started afresh with other groups. When the commandant decided that regular study halls were needed, I became a supervisor and adviser as well as a classroom teacher.

The program was steadily refined. Units in oral communication were added to grammar and composition classes. I was interested in the growing importance given to speech.

One morning a sentence the grammar of which we were discussing contained the word "mules" and a cadet, unable to restrain his curiosity, asked: "What, really, is a mule? How does a mule differ from a horse?" I explained that when a male donkey was crossed with a female horse, the offspring had certain qualities of each parent: the long ears and tufted tail and general sure-footedness of the sire, and the stamina and vigor of the dam. Mules matured earlier than horses, could work longer and harder than horses, but had a reputation for being stubborn.

"Do you always have to start with a donkey and a mare?"

"You sure do. A mule is a sterile hybrid. There are mare mules and horse mules, and their sex organs look normal, but they can't produce offspring."

"What about crossing a female donkey and a stallion?" Obviously these men wanted to get the mule business straightened out once and for all.

"That's possible, but the offspring is not a useful animal. It lacks the good qualities that have made the mule so valuable. If you want a mule, you had better go at it the old-fashioned way."

I could have told them that I had an uncle who owned a prize jack, and a grandfather who had a matched pair of red mules that he would not take $500 for, but I decided I had given them enough information for the time being. From then on, however, they seemed to give me credit for knowing more about either grammar or mules than I really did.

ALONG WITH THE AIRCREW PROGRAM, the University administered an Army Specialized Training Program for especially competent students, filtered out of the regular outfits by examination. As these were the cream of the crop, we felt fortunate to have ASTP sections assigned to us. Months later I heard a rumor that the Army, suddenly running short of manpower, threw groups of these men, who had received more book learning than combat training, onto the Anzio beaches—not a healthy place for anybody.

Before long we were teaching steadily from 7:00 a. m. to 6:00 p. m.—aircrew, ASTP, study hall, civilians.

At 5:00 one afternoon a week, the combined forces staged a parade on the main campus. The bugles sounded, the band played, the flights marched to their places in the massed formation. Commands rang out: present arms, inspect arms, parade rest—the lot. Section leaders bellowed in turn, "Present or accounted for" as the roll was taken, their cries echoing from smaller to larger units until the cumulation of reports reached the parade officer. The flag was lowered, the bugle sounded, the young men and women marched away, the crowd of onlookers dissolved. Another day, another week, had gone by.

The armed forces flooded the campus from the spring of 1943 until the winter of 1944, group following group. I had learned the names of many, many cadets and could greet them when I saw them on campus. We took a deep interest in these young people. Across the nation, other campuses were having similar experiences. Everyone knew that D-Day would be launched sooner or later.[8]

Although I had spent two summers in Citizens Military Training Camp learning close-order drill and the maneuvering of horse-drawn artillery, it was at Syracuse University that I especially appreciated the strong relationship between the military and the art and craft of teaching. At CMTC I had been interested in the officer-teachers and their manuals, visual aids, and instructional procedures; at Syracuse University we taught from military manuals. Everywhere was a mood of urgency: "the difficult we can do at once, the impossible takes a little longer" seemed to apply to education as well as to building tanks and aircraft and to raising food for ourselves and our allies.

64

Teaching Speech: Postwar

FTER FOUR YEARS I had been promoted to associate professor, a move something like going from captain to major. As the University did not issue contracts, I learned of my promotion in the Sunday *Syracuse Herald.*

Occasionally I had received an offer to teach elsewhere; one year I was intrigued by an opening in the Yale Divinity School. I fantasized working with bright young minds entering the ministry and about the contribution I might make to the art of sermonizing and the other kinds of public speeches that a minister makes. Unquestionably one of the best ways to improve church attendance is to provide moving sermons, as demonstrated by the experience of preachers like Henry Ward Beecher, Harry Emerson Fosdick, Billy Graham, and Peter Marshall. I would also have been at the leading edge of efforts to apply principles of communication to situations like interviewing and counseling. But I did not want to move to large, sprawling New Haven, and did not like the idea of teaching an outside or shoulder course in a professional school.

Nor did the inquiry from Bower Aly about returning to the University of Missouri cause any excitement in our Fayetteville home. I did not intend to pursue the matter, but he wrote: "Come and see us. You can visit friends and you don't have to make any advance commitment."

I knew that since May 1940 Missouri had had a new Department of Speech and Dramatic Art. After I had left, my former colleagues had told the dean: "You see what happens when we do not have our own department. We hire someone and soon he resigns and goes to a campus where he can be a professor of speech." I had helped the department more by leaving than by staying. No longer a corner in the Department of English, it could now offer undergraduate major and minor programs and master's and doctor's degrees in speech, theater, speech pathology, and the expanding field of broadcasting.

In Columbia, I interviewed the new dean, zoologist W. C. Curtis, on June 4, 1944. In our initial conversation he dispelled a dozen doubts in a dozen minutes. He was determined to have a strong speech department. When I recalled the former doctrine, "Missouri is a good place to come to and a good place to go from," he labeled it pure stupidity. "Years before the depression, Missouri had a grand tradition. We want to return to that. We are now in the process of making three appointments in the College at full professor level as a step in rebuilding our faculty." I could see that the situation had indeed changed.

Before meeting at a luncheon with deans and professors who had close academic ties to the new department, Curtis told me he was seating me next to the dean of the College of Engineering, who had not shown much interest in my being appointed. I asked questions and found that this dean had been active in the development of the Tennessee Valley Authority. Once I had coached debaters on this topic, so I remembered something about it. At the luncheon, I began by blandly asking him if he had enjoyed his experience with TVA. He talked steadily through the salad and roast beef; whenever he paused I asked him a further question. All in all I uttered perhaps half a dozen sentences. Afterwards, Dean Curtis told me that the engineering dean had spoken enthusiastically about me, adding, "Reid is a fine conversationalist." Somewhere here is a precept, a modest contribution to the art of interviewing.

On the way home, I stopped at Iowa City to visit Craig Baird. At supper we discussed the pros and cons, to move or to stay put, at length. When I went to bed, full of the happenings of the last two days, I felt that I must make a landmark decision. In June the mornings start early, and just as the sun was rising I heard cries and shouts from the street. I lifted my head out of the pillow and tried to make out the words. Newsboys were selling extras: "D-Day! D-Day! Allies Land on Normandy Beaches!"

Back at Fayetteville, Gus and I debated the offer. I talked with dean and chancellor; they made proposals; I made counter-proposals. To meet the proposed rank of full professor was not an unsurmountable problem, but much beyond that they could not go. I have since wondered if buying all that real estate, all of those houses to accommodate military students, had put too crushing a burden on the Syracuse budget. The University had barely survived the war; it had had little time to plan for the future. We decided to return to Missouri.

We brought the barrels up from the basement and one by one Gus packed them. We sold our house but little else, since furniture and other items were impossible to buy except at auctions. Eventually an immense Allied Van drove to our front door; the crew filled it with our accumulations.

We stashed the children in the back end of the Chevy. I had my gas ration book plus the supplementary coupons the local board had allotted for the cross-country trip. Immediately ahead lay a thousand miles of highway that seemed to have been built only for us, so light was the traffic. At the wartime legal speed of 35 miles an hour, we spent four days on the road.

On my last day at Syracuse, I pedaled the seven miles to the Hall of Languages and parked my bike in its usual place. As far as I know, it is still there. I reflected again upon the ancient city bus, hearing its rattling and creaking and grinding gears, and wondered for a last time whether it would make it through the war's final months.

WE WERE SETTLED IN at the University of Missouri when students flocked back to the campus. No one who taught then, wherever he or she was, will forget the experience. Those were golden years of teaching, with mature students, eager to catch up, wanting to learn, willing to work. In all that is said and written about what is wrong with education, little mention is made of those three "w's," wanting, willing, and working.

Only two years before, on a gray, hazy, Syracuse dawn, I had asked my aircrew class: "How many of you will go to college after the war?"

Fundamentally I am a nuts-and-bolts teacher, affixed to my syllabus, but occasionally I steal minutes for a "howgozit" session. Howgozit—the in-flight computation the navigator hands the pilot: here's the destination, here's the mileage still ahead, here's the amount of gas we have left.

So, young fellows, you with the crew cuts, you now with solo time in the air, let's talk about your lifetime goals, the thereafter when the shooting stops. In other words, howgozit.

College? they had responded, unbelievingly. This cotton-picking instructor is out of his cotton-picking mind! When this man's war is over, sir, which will not be for years, sir, we'll be too old for college. Too far behind, sir. We'll not be able to catch up.

I probed, questioned, came at them from other angles, but they stuck to their story. We got just so much gas. We can go just so far.

That's a reason why the campuses were only partly prepared for the glut of students that showed up after V-J day. And then, V-J came sooner than expected; and demobilization of our men and women also came more swiftly than expected. And further: In 1944, after I had talked to the aircrew cadets, the famous legislation to be known as the GI Bill of Rights had been enacted.[1] The bill itself was simple enough. Those who had been in the armed forces would be given a stipend of $50 a month, $75 if they had dependents, plus up to $500 a year for tuition, fees, books, and supplies, to support them while they were enrolled in a college or job-training institution. These benefits would be paid for one year plus an additional period equal to the time the recipient had spent in military service. Later the stipends were increased.

For once, the government was on top of a problem. Wise people, realizing that the end of the war was approaching, had given thought to the serious impact on the nation's social and economic life of suddenly disgorging 16 million men and women into the work force. The job market would be swamped by these hordes of young people, many of whom had been deprived of the normal opportunity to develop vocational skills. Business and industry, in the midst of the transition from wartime contracts to civilian enterprises, would be in no position to hire and train such numbers. And nobody wanted veterans to join the bread line. The Great Depression was still burned into the public memory, and some even recalled the bonus army that had marched on Washington after World War I.

Aside from these economic reasons, the GI Bill was also enacted because Americans were grateful to these men and women, in the forefront of those who liberated the millions living in occupied countries. Thousands of GI recipients came from families that had had no tradition of college attendance. Thousands had been in the bottom segments of their high school classes. No matter, said the colleges and universities, let's admit them, let's give them a chance, let's assume they're mature, or late bloomers who will, with encouragement, succeed. We're not worried about whether or not they actually have a high school diploma. We'll let them start and see whether they can make it. We'll advance them twelve hours of credit in physical education because of their military experience. We'll set up remedial courses, help find tutors, schedule individual conferences, suggest extra reading.

In 1942, total college and university enrollment in the United States was 1,400,000. In 1943, it had dropped to 700,000. By 1944 and 1945 it had approached near normal—1,200,000. But in the next three years it doubled to 2,400,000—of whom more than half were veterans. And a good share of the non-veteran enrollment was made up of those whose education had been interrupted by war work in the factories, on the farms, and elsewhere.

Before the war, an average state university had 4,000 or 5,000 students; during the war its enrollment was cut to half that; after the war the figure grew to 8,000, 10,000, and more. Wartime faculties, even when augmented by returnees, simply could not cope with the exploded enrollment. High school faculties were raided, retired professors were called back to service. Many were hired mainly on promise and potential.

First of all, each student had to find a place to live. University administrators had decreed: If you can give us a local address, we'll register you. We can give you a bed in the gym while you look around, but you must locate a permanent home.

Our local situation reflected the massive, nation-wide housing deficiency that could not be alleviated until seasoned lumber, bricks and cement, hardware, plumbing, and electrical equipment again became available. Vacant apartments were non-existent. So the young people went bell-ringing, in ones, twos, threes. "Do you have a vacant room?" No, no, sorry, no. They rang the bell next door, and at the next. No address, no university education.

Subsequent bell-ringers were more desperate, more persistent. Do you have a room? any space at all? just enough for a bed? Gus finally decided to rearrange the sleeping arrangements of our young ones and rent the smallest bedroom to two GI's, who eagerly agreed to share its double bed, its study table, and its one bathroom at the end of the hall. "Since we're a family of six," she asked, "would you mind taking your showers at the gym?" "Beautiful," they replied. "No trouble at all. At all." And off they flew to complete their registration. Since they could now furnish a mailing address, they could be university students.

We thought we were full up, but still the young men knocked on the door. One pair, more persistent than the others, asked: "Do you have a basement?"

"Yes, but the coal pile is there, and everything is covered with coal dust."

"Can we look at it?"

"Yes, you can look at it, but you'll see it isn't suitable."

They saw the dust, the low ceiling, the poor lighting. They saw the small room with windows and the stool without a lid, but hardly heard me say it had long been disconnected. They exclaimed, "Why, it's a lovely basement!" We said they could move in and try it; they were transported with delight. A mattress on the floor would be just the thing. All week they had been turned down by one householder or another. Their temporary arrangement at the gym was running out. Now they, too, could become university students.

Perhaps we could do better by them than putting a mattress on the floor, but new furniture was impossible to find. Local auction houses (in Columbia we remember Auctioneer Barney Ward) held periodic sales of used furniture, tools, household wares. We located an iron double-decker bunk—frail, shaky, in danger of immediate collapse, but we jammed it into the corner and wired it to the wall. We spared a table and chairs and screwed hooks into the walls for clothes. We swept and hosed the whole basement floor.

We bought wallpaper and a wallpapering outfit and had our first experience of cutting, pasting, and hanging. I recall standing on a stool in a corner of the room, a ten-foot, pasted, doubled over, strip of wallpaper, balanced on the fingers of my upstretched hands, trying to keep fingers from punching through the wet wallpaper, Gus with paste brush in one hand and smoothing brush in the other, and my saying to her, "Can you somehow join me on top of this stool? I need two more hands, although really I think it is impossible to wallpaper a ceiling," and Gus, putting one brush down, and tucking the other under her elbow, responding to the emergency. The toilet, when connected, worked; we located a lid in the junk yard. We bought a small gas heater and ventilated it. Our tenants could come and go through the rear basement entrance. They lived there three years.

One way or another, students found rooms where vacancies had never before existed. Householders, even on silk-stocking streets like Westmount, installed apartments. Everybody had a kindly feeling toward these young people who had helped to liberate Europe and drive back Japan or who had kept the supply lines filled with the tools of war. The University then had only two or three dormitory buildings and no provision for married students.

Married couples, equally determined, also found quarters. If you asked a young husband, "Have you found a place to stay?" he would reply, "Oh, yes, we have a real nice attic room over on Wilson Avenue." Or a young wife would smile, delightedly, "We're so lucky. We live in a basement on Garth Street." Everything is great, we're getting along fine. After the long separation, it was glorious, simply glorious, just to be together—living in an attic, basement, quonset hut, or garage, was secondary.

The three w's were in high gear.

AFTER A STUDENT had an address, the next move was somehow to find enough available courses to fill a schedule. The GI's called the registration procedure "veteran's administration." Classes filled with astonishing speed. A GI came to my office, eager to enroll in public speaking. I checked his program and my schedule. "Don't have a thing."

"I need the course badly. It's required. Can't you squeeze me in anywhere?"

I looked again. "Well, I can give you a seat just inside the door of a Tuesday-Thursday-Saturday section that meets at 7:00 a. m. It is, in fact, now full, but I'll gamble that some one will drop out."

I expected him to turn me down flat—Saturday classes had always been anathema—but his eyes lit up like a rocket flare, and he handed me his form to complete. "God bless you, sir."

Later in the week another GI asked to enroll. By then we had opened up a few spaces. I suggested: "How about 8:00 Monday-Wednesday-Friday?"

"I've got Spanish 1 then, the woman's a real bitch."

"Do you have 11:00 free?"

"Yes."

"Suppose I phone the Spanish department to see if we can get your Spanish moved to 11:00 so you can take speech at 8:00?"

"No, I don't want to change Spanish."

"Okay, but something you said, I don't recall exactly what, made me feel you weren't exactly fond of your Spanish lady."

"She's what I said, whatever that was, but am I learning Spanish! We all are. I'd be crazy to move."

I left his Spanish intact and found another slot for his speech class. When you are next working on your formula for Good Teaching, include this Spanish teacher in your databank.

Classes were jammed and packed. Morale was high. Learning can be one of the world's truly exciting adventures. These older students relearned study habits and developed new ones. Many had not attended any class other than training sessions since their high school commencements. Some had not even formally graduated from high school but were admitted under new, liberal policies. They were, of course, motivated.

They were on the campus because of their own desire to learn. I am trying to contrast the intensity of this desire with that of the average undergraduate and will do so by making the almost-unbelievable declaration that these older men and women studied not only the *assigned* reading but also the *recommended* reading. They stopped at the instructor's desk after class, seeking information on a lecture point. They explained crucial details to one another. The atmosphere was both supportive and exciting.

Our departmental committee scanned applications for teaching assistantships, seeking those who could also take courses toward an advanced degree, now that we were approved for master's and doctor's degrees. Those who had averages of B or better were good risks; if they had done that well as undergraduates, the chances were strong, with their added maturity, they would attain the degree. At times, however, the undergraduate transcript averaged only C, with here and there a dismaying D or F. Normally we would not have encouraged such an applicant to face a course of graduate study at which he or she might not succeed. Those years, however, faculty committees leaned over backwards, feeling that students should have a second or even a third chance.

I have yet to find a professor who does not recall the late 1940s and early 1950s as the peak years of teaching. We worked hard but the rewards were bountiful. Those who met the challenge of that decade felt that teaching was indeed a glorious profession. The few who did not perform at their peak met criticism from these older students. Every hour the stairways were flooded with students going two abreast, squeezing past the pairs coming down. Their scraps of conversation often reflected the excitement of the hour just spent. But I remember an eloquent disclaimer: the young man ahead of me on the stairs, wearing a flight jacket, exclaimed: "That teacher talks like a P-47 coming out of a 6G dive!" I also heard comments even more pungent, since, in general, the older students introduced to the campus a colorful, only slightly laundered, version of GI language.

As shirts and trousers were still almost impossible to buy, the GI's continued to wear military issue. First thing they did, however, was to strip chevrons, stripes, bars, and other insignia from their army shirts, field jackets, and overseas caps. No one wanted to be called by a military title. When a student in a public speaking class was addressed as "captain" by another student, he pleaded: "Don't call me captain. I'm Elbert. I want to forget the war and so do you." Everybody gave him a cheer.

Occasionally we saw an airman who had flown the Burma hump. On the back of his jacket was a message in Chinese, reading something like, "I'm an American, fighting for China. Help me find other Americans." In the event he was shot down, if Chinese natives found him they would know he was a friendly and would help him locate his outfit.

Among our students were former Waacs and other servicewomen. We also had returnees from aircraft or tank assembling lines, shipyards, factories like Chrysler or Douglas Aircraft. I interviewed a student whose age encouraged me to ask, "You've been out of school a while. Why did you come back?"

"I want to wear a blue arm band."

"What do you mean, 'blue arm band'?"

"Right after the war I applied for a job at Ford. The woman at the personnel desk asked me only one question: 'Do you have a college degree?' When I said 'No,' she said, 'Take this card and go to Room 32.' The guy before me had said 'Yes' and she had sent him to Room 207. In Room 32, after the interview, I was assigned a job tending machines. The line was supervised by guys wearing blue arm bands; I learned they were college graduates. I saw right there, the more your education, the better your job. I want to wear a blue arm band."

I worked a schedule out for her, and I hope she got the blue.

The enrollment bulge continued eight years. To meet housing needs, the University steadily acquired army barracks from nearby bases, sawed each one into sections, re-erected the sections on the campus, using some for students, others for classrooms. We called them "T" (for "temporary") buildings, and gave each a number, as "T-100." Small duplexes once occupied by officers were acquired, dismantled, and re-erected. Metal quonset huts appeared. "Faculty housing" and "married student housing," heretofore almost unheard of, sprang up everywhere. So it happened that the concept of University-run housing for married couples came to stay.

When I became department head I could use this temporary housing to recruit graduate students and faculty. I could wire a prospective doctoral candidate: CAN OFFER HALF-TIME TEACHING APPOINT-MENT TWELVE HUNDRED DOLLARS OPPORTUNITY TO TAKE TWELVE HOURS GRADUATE COURSES ALSO THREE-ROOM BARRACKS HOUSING THIRTY DOLLARS MONTHLY. The offer of cheap housing was a lure difficult to resist. We attracted a fine group of graduate students who did much to enhance the reputation of our department. When they took seminars in other areas, they were often outstanding in discussions and presentations because of their added skills in communication. Colleagues in psychology, history, political science, and sociology commented about the fine work that our students were doing in their fields.

In two decades most of the temporary buildings would be razed and replaced with handsome brick structures. Missouri's last T-building disappeared in 1983. Their availability, however, was convenient for these older men and women who wanted to return to the campus and learn a new career.

Eventually half of the eligible veterans—7.8 million men and women—enrolled under the GI Bill. Forced into incredible adjustments, many colleges would have collapsed but for GI Bill revenue. And by the tens of thousands the GI Bill graduates flowed into management, construction, engineering, mechanics, law, medicine, the ministry, other fields. Nearly a quarter of a million became college teachers. The overall effects of the GI Bill were so far-reaching that some have compared its impact on human life with that of the Marshall Plan. (As I write this I have to reflect that most of those GI's are finishing their active careers, and most of their teachers have retired or have passed on.)

Something priceless left us when the last crop of GI's was graduated and we found ourselves again teaching the 16-to-21 group. What they missed was what we missed—the example set by the older students.

SO MUCH OF LIFE hinges on chance encounters.

On a cool, crisp September morning as I walked across the campus, I met Dean Elmer Ellis.

The preliminary greeting was brief. "Can Gus teach mathematics?" he asked. Every department in the College of Arts and Science was short of faculty. Ellis had plunged into the recruiting problem, trying to help department heads recruit staff to teach the flood of students.

"No," I answered. "English, but not math."

"English? She's hired."

Gus's experience was no novelty. I recall want ads seeking teachers: "Don't bother to send us a resume. Just write your name and address on a postcard. We'll get in touch with you." At the time this procedure seemed eminently sensible. Occasionally I could say to a student: "Put a map of the United States on a wall. Throw a dart at it. We'll be able to get you a job where the dart sticks." I did not feel that I was making an unusual statement, and that the student, whatever his or her teaching specialty, could secure an appointment.

Here in the closing decade of the twentieth century we are being told that the demand for teaching staff is increasing so much faster than the supply that we will once again face a critical situation. As we approach the millennium the demand for teachers may again approach that of the late 1940s and 1950s.

Married women, who for years had been spurned because of nepotism rules or because they might displace employed men, were now eagerly sought. One of my graduating seniors told me that she was going to be married right after commencement. She was happy about the prospect, but expressed regret that she would not be able to teach once she was married.

"Where are you going to make your home?" I asked.

"In Cleveland."

"When you get to Cleveland, apply for a job in the city school system."

"But I also lack some of the requirements for a certificate. I still need—" and she mentioned a course or two that she did not have.

"Go ahead and apply. There's every likelihood they'll work out something provisional for you." The Cleveland people eagerly did just that, and she was thrilled to have both home and career.

The president of Ohio State University had told us in a public lecture: "We hired instructors by the scores. One evening I was signing a stack of appointments, and suddenly noted that our baby sitter was being recommended for an instructorship in French. I hated to lose her, but I knew our Romance Language department was desperate for help."

Gus reported to Edward H. Weatherly, then head of the Department of English, and they visited with Harold Y. Moffett, in charge of freshman English. She was given a half-time appointment, which soon became full time, and turned into a lifetime career of teaching English and rhetoric, and of supervising teachers of freshman English.

Our relationship with professors of English was more useful and amiable after we had separated than it had been when we were tied together. We found solid areas of common interest and were freed from each other's eccentricities.

The field of speech, like every other discipline on the campus, had to face head-on the situation of having more students than could be competently taught. Since the problem of teacher shortages was apparent everywhere, the National Association of Teachers of Speech and other learned societies would have to find ways of coping with it.

The Original Gold Card Era

FOR SIX YEARS the University of Missouri campus was to be the administrative center for the National Association of Teachers of Speech. A Columbia firm, Artcraft Press, would print its three major publications, plus those of the American Educational Theatre Association, the Central States Speech Association, and the National University Extension Association. These and scores of lesser printings, like convention programs and membership-drive circulars, would be mailed through the United States postal service in Columbia. Surely this was a major happening, rare in the history of educational organizations. Even the Internal Revenue Service got interested.

Reach for a chair, and read on.

THE FOUR-YEAR-OLD Department of Speech and Dramatic Art had been born in Switzler Hall, which had previously housed the University divisions of Agriculture, Journalism, and Engineering. Each of these had moved on to a better and finer home.

In 1936, before becoming a separate department, our staff had visited the then-empty Switzler. The whole west end of the third floor, to become a cluster of offices for teaching assistants, was a single large area with here and there the big drawing tables that had been abandoned by the engineers. We started the remodeling by partitioning the floor. So many rooms resulted that each professor or instructor could have had a couple, but we were looking ahead to further growth.

The Speech and Hearing Clinic that I had started in 1938 and now a major part of the Department, had a suite of three rooms: two were connected by a one-way mirror so that clinicians could observe a case in progress, yet remain unseen. At the other end of the long hall a large room had been cut in half by a partition, containing a glass window; one room had a microphone, the other a Presto recorder. Now a student could make a speech in one room and be overheard by the rest of the class in the other, and at the same time be record on an aluminum or plastic disc. When he or she had finished, everybody could hear the recording, the speaker being present to share the general amazement. Eventually this area would become the studio for our single course in radio broadcasting. Our list of offerings had more than doubled, with underclass, upperclass, and graduate courses in each of our areas.

We were absolutely, positively, state of the art.

Bower Aly was department head, Director of Forensics and editor of the *Debate Handbook*; its press run of several thousand copies would go to high school and college debaters in each of the forty-eight states. James A. Winans, now retired from Dartmouth College, had a nearby office. I was the sole possessor of the largest single office in the building. From my desk I could look out upon the University's famous columns, and in the winter, when the trees had shed their leaves, could see the big clock on Memorial Tower. Once I contemplated writing Leslie Cowan, business manager of the University, asking him to cut down a few trees so I could have a year-round unobstructed view of the clock, but he was not famous for having a sense of humor so I did not disturb his day. In my lifetime I have made a lot of remarkable decisions like that.

IN DECEMBER 1944 I attended the Chicago convention of the National Association of Teachers of Speech as a new member of its Executive Council. I arrived late at its opening meeting and learned that I had been elected executive secretary. "That's the penalty for being late," the group said.

I asked for time to consult friends. "It's an unparalleled opportunity," said the affirmative. "It'll bring your research to a halt," warned the negative. I knew about Mendel, the Austrian monk who practically invented heredity. "He became abbot of a monastery," a biographer wrote, "and his research ceased." Those who advised me to decline were persuasive, but I accepted anyway; the urge to try something new is difficult to resist. It was a landmark decision, like the one to teach speech instead of English. It was as if someone had said, "Now the country is your campus."

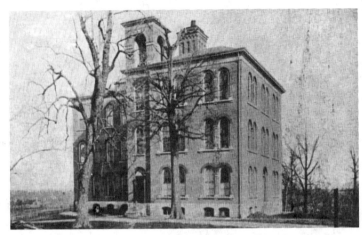

Nineteenth-century picture of Switzler Hall, oldest building on the University of Missouri-Columbia campus. In 1938-39 it became the home of the speech section of the Department of English (the Department of Speech and Dramatic Art was organized May 15, 1940). From 1945 to 1951 the headquarters of the National Association of Teachers of Speech was quartered on the first floor. (*1939 Savitar* [Centennial Issue].)

Joseph F. Smith of the University of Utah, president-elect of the Association, one of the grandest of my professional friends, invited me to his suite to discuss the Association's problems, which had been intensified by the depression and the war. Membership was down. Resources were low. The Placement Service had withered away, yet the demand for teachers of speech would be extraordinary. "And right now," Smith continued, "we do not even have a city for our next convention, much less a hotel." I was well aware of the desperate shortage of hotel accommodations because of wartime traffic: troops and their families on the move, industry and government officials traveling on military business. "Unless you can find us a hotel, we'll have to abandon the 1945 convention." If we had to give up our annual meeting, we would lose an enormous chunk of revenue.

On the train ride home, sitting in the aisle on my suitcase, I reflected on the situation. On the suitcase next to me was a marine, working away on a fifth of bourbon. Already he was glassy-eyed and had half a bottle still to go. I was doubly worried, both about his future and mine. The more I pondered, the glassier my eyes got, even without bourbon; for, although I had staged conventions for the Central States Speech Association in Columbia and Minneapolis, that had been in peacetime when hotels were plentiful and sales managers would wine and dine you and put you up in the Emerald Suite in order to get your convention. Now they would hardly look up from the papers on their desk to say hello to you.

I needed information, and needed it fast. Without a convention and the fees and dues it would attract, we could easily go bankrupt. First no hotel, then no convention, then no Association. I could read the tombstone: "National Association of Teachers of Speech. Founded 1914. Perished 1945. Rest in Peace." All of this in Old English, the type used for funeral notices, wedding invitations, citations, and similar disasters.

I felt much as I had back in northwest Missouri, when I had suddenly got excited about muskrat trapping. I had gone to the local fur buyer and had flooded him with questions. "Where do you go to find muskrats? What kind of traps do you need? What do you use for bait? If you catch a muskrat, how do you skin it?" He told me where and how.

As a preliminary move, I called the secretary of our local Chamber of Commerce. "See Fred Rein of the St. Louis Convention Board. Fred's been in the business longer than any of us." I went to St. Louis and chatted with him; he commented that hotels were currently enjoying an occupancy rate of about 110 percent and didn't really need new business. By 110 percent, Rein continued, the hotel sales managers really meant 110 percent, since they were putting beds in meeting rooms, or in sample rooms, designed for salespeople to display merchandise, or in other rooms not normally used for lodging. Rein advised: "Go to New York and see Howard Dugan, vice-president of the Statler chain. He sits on top of several big hotels and might just accidentally have a spot. Besides, he knows hotel people in the East, where the big establishments are. A point in your favor is that you meet between Christmas and New Year's, which in the hotel racket is the dullest season of the year, because the smart people stay home with their families."

Before going to New York, I made phone calls to Chicago, Cleveland, Detroit, favorite cities of the past. Nothing was available. I was at the end of my rope.

The Statler chain of hotels was known as one that had introduced numerous innovative features for the convenience of guests, like glassine wrappers over drinking glasses and doilies over toilet seats. Dugan extended a cordial invitation to visit him. Seeing him in his burgundy plush office suite, I felt he could work miracles if anybody could. What if professors had burgundy plush offices? Think of the respect they could command.

"Hotel people like conventions of teachers," he confided. "They lend class to our operation. They don't throw much money around but they are not so tough on the furniture. We would love to have your group if we can find a spot."

Dugan was obviously a man of vision who was looking beyond the present to a day when hotels would be glad to have the friendship of a promising young executive secretary. Already I began to feel better.

Dugan phoned Boston, New York, Washington, elsewhere. I could tell by listening to the conversation that every hotel was solidly booked. Next he phoned Buffalo, and found, I think to his surprise, that Buffalo had an open date. Having lived in upstate New York, I knew about Buffalo weather. Especially in late December. I told him I would keep Buffalo in mind but would first investigate other possibilities.

I vividly recall Dugan's friendliness and competence. I have since found that combination of qualities in many successful executives. I also learned about his personal influence ten years later, when, stranded in New York without funds, I walked into the Hotel Pennsylvania and tried to cash a $100 check, a giant sum in those days. Credit cards were then rare. A prudent man might have just one, for, say, Standard Oil. The cashier demurred, saying she did not know me; she did, however, ask if I knew anybody on the hotel staff. "No," I replied, "but I'm a friend of Howard Dugan." She smiled and handed over the money.

Not long afterward, I received a handsome "Gold Card" issued by the Statler system, obviously for its VIP friends, requesting Statler hotels everywhere to extend the bearer every courtesy. I saved it, reflecting that it might help me get a room when the situation was tight. Every traveler has an unshakable belief that no hotel is ever completely full—that somewhere it has an empty room if the desk clerk can be persuaded to surrender it.

In search of sites warmer than Buffalo, I visited The Roosevelt in New Orleans. The sales manager rolled out the red carpet, but when I inquired about facilities for our black members, he fell back on the standard southern position of that day. "We can give them sleeping rooms and serve them in private dining rooms, but cannot let them use elevators, the main dining rooms, or the public rest rooms." "We would like to come to New Orleans," I countered, "but not on those terms."

He was regretful, apart from the thought of losing a lucrative Christmas holiday contract, but pleaded he could make no other arrangements—"that's the way it is." And that was the situation until the civil rights movement of the 1960s.

As a last resort, I tried Cincinnati. It was at least on the edge of the Mason-Dixon line. Nothing was available. Eventually we booked the Deshler-Wallick in Columbus. If we could not go to the South, we would at least get as close as we could.

I WISH I HAD ASKED Father what event the people of his generation would have been sure to remember with such vividness that they could recall where they were and what they were doing when the news of a major event first flashed over the wires. Was the defeat of Bryan and the election of McKinley in 1896 such a date? It was the climax of a bitter, impassioned campaign. The assassination of McKinley? he was a competent but not heroic figure. Perhaps Armistice Day, 1918—even I, then 13, remember that—the enormous bonfire on Main Street in Gilman City, and the men throwing their hats on the blaze.

My generation, young and old, remembers two. One was Sunday, December 7, Pearl Harbor. The other was the sudden death of Franklin Delano Roosevelt, 63, the April before that Columbus convention, and only five months after having been elected to a fourth term by another landslide vote. He and Eleanor seemed always to have lived in the White House.

I learned about Roosevelt's death when it was announced at a meeting of the graduate faculty. For years I had recorded his radio addresses in our speech laboratory in Switzler Hall. Six weeks before he died I had planned to record the address to Congress following the Yalta conference. He began by asking permission to sit down, mentioning it was a lot easier not to have to carry "about ten pounds of steel around the bottom of my legs and also because I have just completed a 14,000-mile trip." This brief reference was his first public comment about his infirmity. We never thought of the President as disabled; he was powerfully built from the waist up, and newspapers, as if by agreement, did not print pictures that showed he was helpless from the waist down.

That night and the next few days radio programs utterly changed their character. Commercials were cancelled, along with comic shows, dramas, and novelties. Instead we heard news bulletins, recollections of the President, and endless somber music. Newspapers also changed their tone; a few, for a day or so, cancelled advertising; all printed endless columns about the Roosevelt years.

Gradually I became aware that little was being written or spoken about Roosevelt's genius as a *speaker*. He was considerably the most eloquent president since Lincoln, and I am not forgetting Teddy Roosevelt nor Woodrow Wilson. Late the next night after FDR's death I uncovered my Underwood and wrote a feature about his speechmaking, and early next morning took it to the *Columbia Missourian* office. I wrote, in part:

> Roosevelt's language was simple, direct, vivid. He addressed us as "My friends" or "My fellow Americans." He pledged a "New Deal." He told us we had "nothing to fear but fear itself." He advised us not to "hide our money under the mattress." He urged us to "quarantine the aggressor nations." He scorned those who "plunged the dagger into the back of a neighbor." He pledged that he would redeem the "date which will live in infamy." He wanted us to become "good neighbors." He used simple illustrations, such as the analogy of the constable who could not arrest the burglar until the town council had met. . . .
>
> It is no accident that his speeches are memorable. He revised them again and again. In the library at Hyde Park is a series of manuscripts showing twenty-two revisions of a single speech—each revision more specific, more vivid. . . .
>
> [Roosevelt had] a calm, quiet, conversational voice, but it had a ringing quality. We have only to think of 1933, when the banks were closed; of 1939 and 1940, when the world was aflame; of 1941, when he told the largest audience that ever listened to a radio that we would avenge Pearl Harbor.

Decades have passed and we still have not had a president who spoke so well at press conferences, during campaigns, at national conventions, before Congress, and in all kinds of broadcasting situations, from a fireside chat that restored our confidence in the nation's ability to survive a depression, to a solemn declaration of war that heightened our determination to overcome disaster and to win the final victory. Millions of people around the world, in news reels and on radio, saw and heard the art of communication as practiced by a master: the clear but often-moving language, the facial expression, the shaking or nodding or wagging the head, the organ tones.

Many who do not remember the death of Roosevelt do remember a similar event: the assassination of John F. Kennedy. They, too, remember where they were and what they were doing when the news that "the President has been shot" was broadcast—this time by network television as well as by radio.

MUCH OF MY HOTEL SEEKING occurred during the early months of 1945, before I actually assumed the office of executive secretary. On July 1 a van arrived from Detroit, bearing the worldly goods of the Association.

Dean W. C. Curtis was pleased to have the office on the campus and through his intercession the Association became a part of the administrative system. I had many conversations with Purchasing, Personnel, and Buildings and Grounds. We were authorized to purchase office supplies through the University purchasing office. We could requisition Buildings and Grounds to build cabinets for us. We could acquire secretarial and clerical help through Personnel. Since about that time I inherited the post of department head, I needed all the help I could get.

The office equipment of the Association reflected depression-time and wartime stringencies. It owned two loose-jointed Underwood typewriters; a paleolithic Addressograph for printing addresses on envelopes; a desk and two chairs; 5,200 issues of back issues of journals; a cigar box containing paper clips, 3-cent stamps, two typewriter erasers, a bottle of Skrip, pens and pen points, stubby pencils. Eventually items like these would become collectibles and displayed in a museum. Part of the reason for the meager equipment was that it had been impossible to buy new office equipment during the war, even if the Association had had the money.

A single four-drawer filing cabinet held correspondence, advertising contracts, and bills and receivables. The Placement Service, on which we would need to count so heavily in locating teaching staff, had less than a drawer-full of folders, many of them obviously not up to date. In all, the Association had only enough stuff to cover a 9 x 12 rug. With slightly more than $1,000 in the bank we could barely meet our first month's bills. Our annual operating budget was $18,000.

I quickly found that the duties of the executive secretary were not well defined. No "Manual of Instruction" accompanied the office. During the first few weeks when a new problem arose, I would call Cortright, or members of the Finance Committee such as Alan Monroe of Purdue or Clarence T. Simon of Northwestern, or sage friends like W. Norwood Brigance of Wabash College. Mainly the talk helped clarify the problem but when the response so often boiled down to "use your own judgment," I decided to do just that. I had the general directive to work for the welfare of the members; I invariably consulted with others involved, for example a journal editor or a program chairperson; otherwise, I did what had to be done.

I had held my new title only a short time when I received a bill for $1,500 for printing an issue of the *Quarterly Journal of Speech*. (In the 1990s this budget item exceeded $10,000.) I was astonished, then appalled. The Wisconsin printer, who specialized in academic journals, insisted the sum was correct. I thereupon walked across the street to talk to Heath Meriwether, proprietor of Artcraft Press, about doing our printing. For years he had printed the *Debate Handbook*; he had also printed the program and publicity materials for the Central States convention in Columbia. I felt enterprising, carrying on a high-powered discussion with a prospective new printer when I couldn't even pay the current bill of the old printer. I also felt I was drawing freely from my years of growing up in a newspaper office. I knew the trade vocabulary, sacred and profane. I was familiar with type faces, the point system, press runs.

First we discussed the shortage of book paper, since an effect of the war was the undependable supply from the mills. It would be embarrassing to shift printers and then discover the new printer could not even secure paper. Meriwether suggested that if the Association could invest in a whole carload, the supply would be more dependable. I gasped when he mentioned *carload*; as a kid I had spent hours playing around boxcars and thought of them as having immense capacity. He, however, did not have the capital required for purchasing and storing. I did not get around to telling him that I was not exactly over-capitalized.

Meriwether noted that labor costs would escalate; we agreed to include a provision in our agreement covering possible increases. I showed him journal articles that contained phonetic symbols, mathematical equations, Greek words. He looked through his Linotype style books and decided that one way or another he could locate what was needed. Much of what was needed, however, we told each other, was made out of brass, a strategic metal, and the Mergenthaler Linotype Company might be fresh out of Greek sigmas or phonetic symbols. Our bold discussion must have been typical of others that were taking place in the postwar era. Even so both of us felt that somehow we could manage the unknowns, the uncertainties, the contingencies.

Our contract was a simple memorandum, to which we made verbal alterations as occasions arose. Over the years we never had a dispute or a misunderstanding. I called the two journal editors, Karl R. Wallace of the University of Virginia and Russell Wagner of Cornell University, described the pros and cons of the situation, and found them willing to share the risk of shifting printers.

When I asked Banker Larry Sapp, my friend and neighbor, if he could loan us $10,000, his answer was succinct: "We do not know your organization but we do know you and Gus and if you will both sign the note you can have the money." We both signed; we had never before borrowed money.

After much phoning and telegraphing, Meriwether located a mill that could sell us the paper; the quality was fair, but acceptable. Not for three more years would paper mills be able to achieve normal peacetime inventories. The saving to the Association was substantial, and, more to the point, we received better service from our new printer. One way or another we squeaked through month by month and issue by issue. Twice we ran completely out of paper; once when an edition of *Speech Monographs* was due. Meriwether got on the phone and managed to locate a supply of a somewhat inferior grade. I mailed a sample to Wagner and said we could go to press with *Monographs* now, or delay the issue and get something better later. He asked a chemist to test the sample for acidity and was told it would eventually self-destruct, but not right away, so he decided he would rather get the issue printed than delay it indefinitely.

WE CALLED THAT 1945 CONVENTION at the Deshler-Wallick a "Reconversion Conference," to indicate that victory was in sight and we were beginning to prepare for peace. The day before the convention began, a disastrous sleet storm lashed the Midwest and attendance was severely reduced. I still remember the thin lines we had registering for rooms and later for admission badges. I made the rounds of morning programs; a few section meetings failed to materialize at all; in two instances the chairpersons simply joined forces and telescoped their programs. The second day's meetings were better attended, but the situation was discouraging. We were lucky to have the five hundred people who managed to arrive, most of them late.

As I had given the sales manager a highly optimistic story when I had booked the hotel, I hunted her up to express my regret that we were making such a poor showing. "You must have a lot of empty rooms," I said.

"Well, we did have 150 cancellations."

"That's simply terrible," I ventured, sincerely regretful.

"You know, it's really not too bad. We are full up. We had overbooked just exactly 150 people."

WILBUR GILMAN, Bower Aly, and I had been working on a manuscript of a public speaking text, and had engaged a suite in the St. Louis Statler where we could hole up for a weekend to make basic decisions. Gilman and Aly were efficient, no-nonsense men who planned meticulously, in detail, and in advance. Aly's letter to the Statler had clearly stated the time of our arrival and our need for a suite that would accommodate the three of us. Aly certainly must have received a confirmation, and maybe even had reconfirmed the reservation, leaving nothing to chance. Arriving on schedule at The Statler, we were told by the clerk that no suite was available. My colleagues were firm, then insistent, then indignant, but the clerk could promise only scattered single rooms for each of us.

Standing at one side, listening, I suddenly thought of the Gold Card that Howard Dugan had given me months before and that I always carried on trips. This must be the sort of emergency for which it was designed. Without saying anything, I unobtrusively placed it on the counter.

The clerk noticed it instantly. "Are you with this party, sir?" he asked. Obviously his problem now had suddenly acquired major dimensions.

"Yes, I am. We did request a suite."

He picked up my card and disappeared behind a partition. We could hear him agonize to his superior: "There's a Gold Card bastard out there and he needs a suite." After whispered dialog, the supervisor himself appeared. Totally ignoring my impressive associates, he addressed himself to me: "We are terribly, terribly sorry about this oversight. We will make you as comfortable as we can tonight in single rooms. In the morning, the very minute a suite is available, we will send our staff to help you move. I cannot tell you how embarrassed we are, but this is the very best we can do." Gilman and Aly were subdued by his explanation and accepted the arrangement.

Next morning three bellhops speedily moved us to a parlor with lounge chairs, thick-piled carpet, paintings on the walls. A basket of fruit was on the table. The three bedrooms each had bath, telephone, and radio. We were mollified and did a week-end's hard work.

When we checked out, Gilman and Aly paid only single-room rates; my bill was complimentary. Suddenly I realized what it meant to hold a Gold Card. Later I learned that Gold Cards were issued only to a select list, and that, throughout the chain, managers were required to extend every possible, conceivable courtesy to the holders, any one of whom might be an individual (like me?) who could send thousands of dollars worth of business to the organization. To offend a holder in the slightest degree might cost a manager his job. And, no doubt, managers often faced trying requests from this influential group.

Before long, this story became known to professors of speech everywhere. Even in the 1990s are a few who know me as the original, genuine, Gold Card bastard.

Except for one memorable occasion, I made no personal use of the card. The manager of the St. Louis Statler had repeatedly invited me to be a guest even though he knew I could not bring him a convention since his hotel did not have enough meeting rooms to accommodate us. "Come and spend a weekend with us," he would say. "Bring your family." One summer I accepted his offer. When the six of us arrived, we were shown to a choice suite with its grand piano and other lush furnishings, and, this time, with a television and a bottle of wine as well as a basket of fruit. The manager himself came along to see that everything was in order.

The youngsters, ages 16 and downward, were impressed. Nothing their father had ever done so thrilled them as the simple fact that he could command the use of sumptuous quarters like these. They inspected all the rooms, sprawled over all the beds, used all the bathrooms. They saw a Cardinal baseball game on the suite's TV—their first exposure to this new medium—and, that evening, a live Browns game featuring that fantastic black pitcher, Satchel Paige— memorable also for saying, "Don't look back, someone might be gaining on you."

When my term as executive secretary expired, my Gold Card was not renewed but was passed on to my successor. That brought me face to face with another reality in the business world: when you are shorn of power and influence, your perquisites fade, fade away.

THE OFFICIAL HISTORY of the Association has this sentence: "*Speech Monographs* was a single-issue volume through 1947 . . . since 1950 it has been a quarterly publication of the Association."

Let me call upon the patrician art of enhancement to expand that statement.

Those years we mailed each copy of *The Quarterly Journal of Speech* and *Speech Monographs* in an envelope, the whole staff gathering around to stuff the envelopes and tie up the packages. The Post Office Department then required that individual copies—"singles," we had called them back in the country newspaper office I had grown up in—of newspapers or magazines had either to be wrapped or put in envelopes. We mailed *Monographs* at third-class rates, putting a stamp on each envelope. By contrast, the *Quarterly Journal* was mailed second class, at a more favorable rate and without all that stamp licking, since the postoffice weighed the bundles and calculated a bulk rate that we could pay by check. We became so weary of affixing stamps that I consulted the postmaster about a second-class mailing permit for *Monographs* and learned we could have a permit only if we published at least four times a year. As we needed more pages anyway for our growing volume of research, we decided to publish quarterly. Editor Lester Thonssen of the College of the City of New York was elated with the decision, which started with the not very scholarly reason that we hated to lick stamps. Obviously I write this footnote to history in confidence, "eyes only"; it is not something you want noised around. Thonssen therefore became the first to edit a quarterly *Monographs*.

As a boy I had grown up with printing machinery and was eternally fascinated by mechanical devices. Gadget shops and Madison Avenue became prosperous mainly because of customers like me. Soon we had a gizmo that slit open the envelopes in the morning mail. And about this time I learned about Pitney-Bowes postage meters and leased an ingenious machine that not only eliminated stamps but that would also seal envelopes. It was the first on the campus; when the secretaries in the University business offices learned about it, they asked if they could use it, persuading their bosses to pick up a share of the rental tab. I was also a natural to buy one of the first electric typewriters, which led to a Robotyper, to be introduced later, and a new and faster machine for addressing journal envelopes.

EACH FALL the Association had published a *Directory*, with a geographical feature that also listed institutions and the members connected with each. We had struggled through the 1945 and 1946 editions, a slow, tedious job of typing a long list of names from the 3x5 cards that constituted our subscription records. The staff would start typing the list of names in October, and by the time the job was finished many of the names had been dropped, many more had been added, and still others had changed addresses.

One noon I left home after a hurried luncheon, and started the slow, 15-minute walk back to the campus. What should we do about the *1947 Directory*? The publication had never been so popular with the membership as one might think. For the first block I reflected that if we just threw the project into the Missouri River, we would save ourselves a lot of trouble, and a lot of money for the Association. Then I reflected: What if we added more information about each member? Instead of the usual simple entry such as:

WEBSTER, Noah, Compendium Lane, Goshen, N.Y.

we printed something like:

WEBSTER, Noah, Instr. of Rhetoric, Goshen Academy, Goshen, N.Y.; B.A. Yale, 1778; admitted to the bar, 1781.

And then added a list of professional interests, such as:

Forensic rhetoric, lexicography, orthography, etymology . . .

followed by the address.

Arriving at the office, I discussed the idea with the women who had been doing the typing. Though it seemed too late in the year to start such a venturesome project, we decided to go ahead with it anyway. We drafted forms to be mailed to the membership to collect the new information. We calculated the number of lines per entry and the number of additional pages that the *Directory* would require. We got estimates from Artcraft Press, called members of the Finance Committee, and got the green light.

The new information about each member would include graduate and undergraduate degrees and schools, with dates, and notations of special interests such as public speaking, speech pathology, or theater. Surely data like these would have historical as well as current value. We mailed information blanks and as an afterthought enclosed a membership renewal form, hoping to collect dues in October as well as at the annual December convention: "Pay now so that your name will be in the new *Directory*." As another afterthought we added the date of expiration, so each member could see where he or she was paid up to.

In a few days the blanks began to come back. Some members, having been asked their specialties, wrote in a dozen, plus a list of their publications. Obviously we could not print everything submitted. We had to retype practically everything.[1]

But how the cash poured in! Nearly every envelope contained money. Our bookkeeper, a GI agriculture student's wife, started working evenings, as did our chief compiler, wife of an instructor who was a GI. In the whole office we suddenly felt as if we were working for a Going Concern. One evening I told Gus and the children, "We've got $5,000 in the bank!" Their faces lit with delight and incredulity, only to droop when they realized the head of the house was just talking shop.

The final form of each entry looked like this:

Kelly, Wilma, Asst. Prof., Dir. of Debate, Manchester College, N. Manchester, Ind. B.A. Indiana State Teachers Col. '31, M.A. Northwestern U. '35, addl. sums. U. of Wisconsin '36, '38, Ph.D. Purdue U. '48. Pub. spk., sp. educ., radio; minor Eng. 23 S. Diana St., Manchester, Ind.

Eventually the copy was prepared and the long job of proof reading began. The opportunities for making mistakes were fearful, working as we did with so much detailed copy written in longhand. Came the day when the *Directory* was printed, put in envelopes, stamped, and mailed. I thought to myself, "We must be prepared to be blasted by a hundred critical letters." Instead, we received no criticism at all. If we had made mistakes, nobody seemed to mind. The new *Directory* was half again as thick as its predecessors, and members were pleased with it. Each entry became, in fact, a four-line biography. Of course the basic rule that everybody grows up with in a country weekly is that people like to see their names in print. And for weeks the monotonous flow of cash and checks continued. Unexpectedly, our income increased, and also became less cyclical.

When mid-spring came we sent out a second letter to the membership, announcing that we planned to print a supplement to the *1947 Directory*. We wanted to enlist the interest of those who had enrolled too late for inclusion in the principal volume. Again we received a flow of blanks and cash, and in due course distributed a 16-page *Supplement*. Additional income means, to an educational organization, funds for stimulating teaching, research, and publication.

TEN YEARS EARLIER the Association had renewed its interest in starting a third journal, this one for the classroom teacher. Gilman had been head of a committee to collect opinions, and had secured letters from fifty leaders in the field as to the wisdom of such a publication. These he had edited and had printed in a pamphlet. The Council, however, had decided against the enterprise; memories of the Great Depression were still too close at hand.

As one faced with the necessity of keeping the organization solvent, I knew we must have additional sources of revenue, and thought again about launching this new journal. At the next Council meeting I proposed that we undertake what I called *The Speech Teacher*. Opposing arguments were persuasive; some doubted that we could get enough good material; others hated to add to an already tight budget. Still, we thought that if we could develop a circulation of 1,000 copies we would break even. At the meeting came a moment when everyone was talked out. In this impasse, James H. McBurney, dean of the School of Speech at Northwestern University, asked: "Do you think we can finance this?" I was sure we could. "Well, then, let's do it." Dallas Dickey of the University of Florida was its first editor; he and his staff liked the title, *The Speech Teacher*, and in January 1952 the first issue appeared.

As it happened, my successor as executive secretary, Orville A. Hitchcock of the University of Iowa, had the heavy responsibility of financial and technical details, but he got the new publication under way handsomely, thanks largely to his energetic promotion. In two years it had a circulation of more than 2,000, of which 175 were libraries. Other libraries were added as soon as the librarians were convinced the new journal was here to stay. That total was not so impressive as the 1,263 libraries which then took *The Quarterly Journal of Speech*, but it was a good start.[2] *The Speech Teacher* continues in the present decade as *Communication Education*.

Our printer, Heath Meriwether, established a close personal relationship with each of the twenty or more editors under whom he served—or, as each of them would proudly put it, who served under him. He

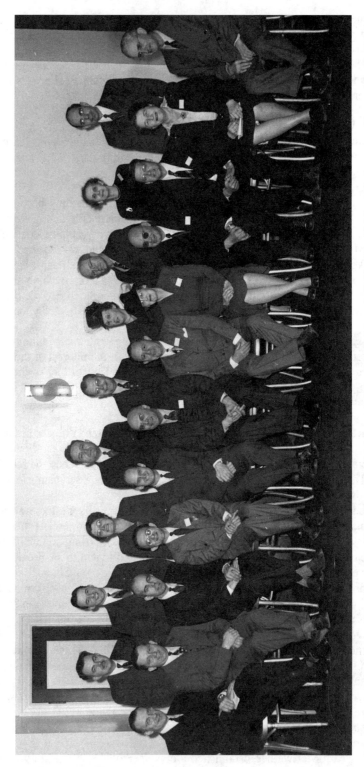

Members of the Executive Council, 1946, are (seated from left to right) Joseph F. Smith, P. Merville Larson, Rupert L. Cortright, Valentine B. Windt, Karl F. Robinson, W. Hayes Yeager, W. Norwood Brigance, Magdalene Kramer, Robert West, Loren Reid, Mabel F. Gifford, and Andrew T. Weaver. Standing from left to right are Franklin H. Knower, Paul D. Bagwell, Gladys L. Borchers, Bower Aly, Joseph F. O'Brien, Ruth Thomas, Karl R. Wallace, Hazel Abbott, and Kenneth G. Hance.

attended our conventions and met authors and officers. No one could adapt more flexibly to deadlines. If an editor had a last minute correction, Heath could manage it; in fact, he could reset the lines himself and insert them in the galleys or pages. He could pronounce "Winans" and spell "Thonssen"; he knew who was "Harold" and who was "Herold"; he could distinguish between "Jeffery" as in "Auer" and "Jeffrey" as in "Robert"; he knew that "Giles" was pronounced with a soft *g*; he learned the subtle differences among the phonetic symbols that bobbed up occasionally in articles. He called a hundred people by their first names. If I had made no other decision in 1945 than to launch a deal with Heath, I would have earned my stipend ten times over.

Meriwether's reputation spread so rapidly that soon he was printing *The American Educational Theatre Journal* and *The Central States Speech Journal*, as well as continuing to print the *Debate Handbook*. He printed Winans' book, *Daniel Webster and the Salem Murder*—Webster was Dartmouth College's most distinguished alumnus, and Winans had taught there—and half a dozen textbooks for me. If I took copy for *Speaking Well* to him in February, he would have it printed and bound by April. As I have said, for two decades Columbia was the center for the publication of speech journals. When Heath retired in 1974, the 60th anniversary of the Association, he was an honored guest at the anniversary luncheon: tributes, standing ovation—everything but fireworks and release of balloons and doves.

For me an amazing fact was that he managed all that typesetting with only two Linotypes.

I am not overlooking Heath's wife, Agnes, who was an undeclared dividend to all of us. She was bookkeeper, proofreader, and expediter. Her efficiency did not detract from her continual good nature. You cannot write the history of our discipline for the four decades after the depression without the names of Agnes and Heath.

DURING THE SIX YEARS that the Association office was in Columbia, I employed perhaps twenty women, most of them wives of servicemen who were continuing the education that had been interrupted by the war. These bright, attractive women typed correspondence, managed the Placement Service, filled orders, mailed circulars and journals. For $125 a month, the prevailing scale at University offices, they worked full time, 8:00 to 5:00. They could have earned more working for an attorney or insurance company, but they liked being on the campus. At noon they could join their husbands for a brown bag lunch, chatting an hour before returning to work. The wives enjoyed each other's company and took a keen interest in what the Association was doing. One of them said: "Here I was, living in a trailer with little to do, and nobody to talk to until my husband came home, and now I have an interesting job with these other girls, and besides can earn a bit."

Moreover, a few of them promptly got pregnant. My colleagues, envious at my association with these likeable women, began to make remarks. The women, however, blamed their new condition on the Robotyper, a machine a little larger than two two-drawer filing cabinets side by side. You would put your electric typewriter on top of it, make certain adjustments and attachments, and on the typewriter compose a letter that you wanted to send to a number of people—same letter but different names and addresses—and your letter would be punched out by something like a player-piano roll. The Robotyper would merrily type the same letter over and over, stopping only long enough for its attendant to type a new name and address and to roll in a new letterhead. Thus it happened that whenever a wife came to work and made an Announcement, the chorus was, "Well, the Robotyper has been at it again." Rossum's Universal Robot Factory would have been amazed by what was going on in Switzler Hall. And what Rossum could have done with the miracles achieved by computers, I have avoided thinking about.

Later we would work with the Boomers from the Great Baby Boom. Here it was, booming before our very eyes.

We lived in the days when we mailed a December journal on or before December 1, a February journal on or before February 1. Now academic journals are called, vaguely, "winter issue" or "spring issue" and mailed at irregular intervals. Letters received on a Monday had a reply in the mail by Tuesday. On occasion the husbands, coming at 5:00 to collect their wives, would find them still busy on an envelope-stuffing job, and would pitch in and help so we could get the sackfuls to the postoffice and thus meet our own deadlines.

I could never have met my teaching and other responsibilities, and at the same time those of the Association, without the unflagging help of all these young women.

ONE OF THEM, Barbara, was a speech major who had planned to teach, but had abandoned that plan to stay in Columbia with her husband, John, while he studied for a degree. When I found she could type, I employed her and assigned her to the Placement Service. Together we surveyed the odds and ends of credentials, prepared by the candidates themselves, often poorly typed and sometimes handwritten. We overhauled the system and began to type credentials in the office, to give them a professional touch. When we circulated the membership both to recruit new candidates and to locate vacancies, our mail doubled and tripled. Barbara was an ideal manager. Her being a speech major helped, and she had, in addition, genuine administrative talent.

Because superintendents and department heads over the country were adding staff, we wondered about setting aside a special room at the upcoming Chicago convention at The Stevens so that prospective employers and candidates could schedule interviews. No such arrangement had ever existed; in fact, some members thought that to encourage job hunting at a convention would make it too much like a slave market. But since the demand for teachers was phenomenal, we went ahead. The mechanics would be simple: a bulletin board on which to post vacancies, an assignment sheet on which interested candidates could sign for appointments, and a supply of desks and chairs. An important step was to notify schools and colleges—chairpersons, deans, superintendents, applicants—so that the plan would get ample publicity.

I asked Barbara if she and John would go to Chicago, be on duty during the convention to schedule interviews and in other ways to help job seekers and employers. I offered to pay their expenses. "You will have three busy days, like from 8:00 a. m. to 6:00, but your evenings will be free," I added.

Over lunch she discussed the proposal with John and they accepted. "We got married and came directly here, so we didn't have time for a honeymoon," she confided. "We decided a Chicago trip would be a nice honeymoon."

In the weeks before the convention the staff mailed out programs and prepared registration materials. Now we also had to devise forms for our new plan of interviewing and have Meriwether print them. We finished these tasks none too soon. Later indications were that this convention would be twice as large as any before it. Since Barbara and John would arrive at The Stevens before I would, I told her: "Because we sometimes have a last-minute crisis, I'd like you to leave a note in my box with your room number, so if I need emergency help I'll know where to find you. I may not arrive until late."

Sure enough, the Wabash Bluebird was jammed with Christmas travelers and I did not reach the hotel until midnight, bone weary from having had to stand up for half the trip and shepherd huge suitcases filled with convention material that I could not trust to overloaded express facilities. To my surprise I found, at the hotel registration desk, three of my friends, grim and irritable because they had been unable to get rooms. "Now that our cosmic executive secretary is here, obviously in full control," they said, with an edgy irony, "we can get this tangle untangled."

"We'll get you rooms right away," I said, with an assurance that was obviously unconvincing.

The clerk shoved a card at me and I filled it out. When he saw my name, his manner changed. "Professor, we've been expecting you. We're looking forward to a fine convention."

"Thank you, but we've got a small problem right now. Here are the president of our Association, the editor, and the chairman of our finance committee, the big wheels who run the show; they tell me they've been unable even to get the rooms that they had reserved."

Suddenly he became eager to please. He knew a Gold Card bastard when he saw one.

"We'll get right at it." He disappeared, came back with a handful of keys, handed each of us a key, and banged the desk bell. In minutes, rooms, guests, and bellboys were paired off. I felt vastly relieved. I had put on quite a display of influence. My friends were even more relieved.

As we all turned to go, the clerk called after me: "Professor, here's a note that was left for you."

We were already ten steps away. "Read it," I said, grandly. "It's probably from the mayor, offering us the key to the city."

He started to bring the note to me, but I waved him back. "Go on. Read it." He glanced at it, gulped, but complied. "I'm in Room 2772. Barbara."

I am not sure whether my status with these great men of the Association rose or fell, but next day they archly made inquiries about Barbara. Relieved to have the opportunity, I took them to the large room where she and John were working, and introduced them. She wondered why she was the center of attention. John wondered even more.

The convention was an unprecedented success; hundreds there had not attended a national meeting since before the war; more than 1,200 registered, our largest number up to that time. Barbara and John worked so steadily and were such a help both to appointing officers seeking talent and to applicants eager for jobs, that the plan of scheduling interviewing worked even better than we had planned. Other organizations heard about it and wrote us for details.

Wartime couples had all sorts of honeymoons and often none at all, but Barbara and John's was one they would cherish. The Association collected so many extra and unexpected dollars from placement fees that it, too, could cherish the arrangement.

MONTHS LATER. Atop my desk blotter was an envelope bearing the return address of the Internal Revenue Service. My heart speeded to 100 beats a minute, even though the envelope was clearly for me as executive secretary, not as industrious teacher, devoted husband, and loving father.

"Dear Professor," it began, "our records show you have not filed a complete return for the National Association of Teachers of Speech. You seem to be liable for a manufacturers' tax in accordance with the calculations on the attached sheet. Please arrange for an interview."

The amount involved was $560, a formidable sum, and one which the Association would be embarrassed to produce at this time of year. We were still in hock for a carload of paper.

At the interview, sitting across the table from the IRS auditor, I expressed my astonishment at the letter, insisting I was not a manufacturer.

Auditors do not cave in easily. "Do you employ more than three people?"

"Yes. In all, six. And then there's me."

"Do you sell a manufactured article?"

"You might call *The Quarterly Journal of Speech* a manufactured article. We make it and sell it."

"You charge for it?"

"Yes. We have paid subscribers."

"And does this manufactured article contain advertising?"

"It does. Thirty pages an issue. Sometimes forty or more."

"For which you collect money?"

"That's correct."

"Well, then, you are a manufacturer and you are liable for a manufacturers' tax, as we said in our letter."

I looked at him with honest blue eyes and adjusted the muscles of my face to show serenity and integrity. "No, I'm not a manufacturer."

"Not a manufacturer? If you're not a manufacturer, what are you?"

"I'm a humanitarian."

Here was a term he had not met in training school. "What's a humanitarian?"

"A humanitarian is a person who does good for people. My Association serves teachers who helps young folks read poetry and drama, make speeches, and learn skills like conversing and interviewing. Some of our teachers help youngsters who stutter or have other speech difficulties. The journal we publish contains articles that help teachers do these things better. The advertisers are firms that sell books and classroom supplies. I do not intend to make a profit, though I do need to make expenses. The University gives me a free office, because it realizes I am a person who helps teachers. That is why I say I am a humanitarian."

He started to ask a question but didn't. "We'd better see my supervisor, Mr. Spaulding, about this."

The auditor reviewed the situation for Mr. Spaulding, who asked questions and then concluded: "The professor is correct. He is clearly a humanitarian and not a manufacturer. We can drop the claim against him."

I was relieved at this happy outcome. I guess I do not need to explain why I remember the name of Spaulding whereas I have forgotten every other IRS auditor I have had to face. I hope he knows he has the appreciation of grateful humanitarians everywhere.

NO ONE KNOWS the full burdens of an association as intimately as the executive officer. Committees and councils meet occasionally and correspond; the executive secretary, the managing director, can never let go.

I would steal away from home on Saturdays and even Sunday afternoons and go to the office, thinking: "I will clear this desk of its accumulation, so that, come Monday, I'll be caught up." This activity became known among my friends as "Reid's Illusion." It has similar names in the homes of other master-executive types. The illusion was snapped every Monday when mail and telegrams and long distance calls brought a fresh supply of problems.

We also had a small but steady flow of complaints. Four advertisers wanted a cover page but we had only two. Library subscribers had failed to receive Vol. XXXIII, No. 3. An Ohio member had been promised a $4 room at the convention hotel and had had to pay $5.

A professor of oral interpretation was miserable because the national office was not working diligently enough to advance his specialty. In fact, he berated us severely. One day, however, he wrote in a more pleading tune: since his health would no longer allow him to endure midwestern summers and winters, could I help him get a position farther south? I had just had an inquiry from a southwestern university, and mentioned (just barely) my persistent complainer. Amazingly, he got the job. Soon after I received from him, not a thank-you note, but another growl: "In your new *Directory* you refer to 'oral interpretation' as 'oral interp.' This abbreviation is degrading. 'Interp indeed! Why can't you spell it out?'"

As I have explained, each *Directory* entry included the member's specialty, abbreviated: "sp path," for example, for "speech pathology." This professor of pub spk tossed the complaining letter into the wstebskt. Some folks you can never please.

For a while an angry letter would dim my day, but the human system has its own defenses and before long I was taking each upbraiding in stride.

As the amount of cash flowing into Switzler Hall began to double and triple, I felt we should have an outside audit and also that we should be incorporated. An audit would protect the integrity of the executive secretary, whoever he was, and incorporation would limit liability in the event of a legal misadventure. I took these matters to the Council, who thought neither of these actions was necessary, but to humor me they let me proceed. A local certified public accountant, then at the dawn of his career, did the auditing. He could tell us at the end of our fiscal year what our assets and liabilities actually were. He also showed us that we had a "net worth"; and that if we were a dime off at the end of any day, we could make a simple bookkeeping entry instead of wondering if it had rolled under the desk and moving the desk to make sure. A local attorney prepared papers for the office of the secretary of state that showed we were an educational—make that "humanitarian"—organization, operating for the general welfare.

Not more than ten people in the nation know offhand that the National Association of Academic Teachers of Public Speaking, which became the National Association of Teachers of Speech, which became the Speech Association of America, which became the Speech Communication Association, was incorporated under the laws of the magnanimous, large-hearted, state of Missouri. The Charter of Incorporation is one of the few tangible remains of the Association's six-year sojourn in Columbia.

Convention Hotels and Other Perils

A S ALREADY SUGGESTED, an Executive Secretary visits many hotels in search of a suitable convention site. Although we wanted to meet in different parts of the country, in the 1940s and 1950s, in order to accommodate all the organizations meeting with us—the American Speech Correction Association, the American Educational Theatre Association, the National University Extension Association, and the American Forensics Association—we were limited to the largest cities and often to the largest hotel in the city. We also needed to contract with hotels well in advance of the convention date. At first they would not plan more than a year or two ahead, but they were beginning to open up their reservation books for later scheduling. Before long we were booked three years ahead; my successors increased the span to five.

After collecting hotel brochures and information about theater and other local attractions, I then visited each promising hotel, was greeted by the sales manager, and given a tour of the facilities.

After an experience or so I learned to anticipate contingencies. Long after an agreement had been reached, a sales manager might phone: "Professor, would you mind giving us back the Susquehanna Room from noon to 2:00 on Tuesday? Our Rotary Club is planning a special program for their wives . . . they're regular customers . . . yes, I know, we promised you all our meeting rooms, but this is a special situation ." So I would offer to see what we had booked that hour, and get on the phone to the people involved. One learns to ask for an abundance of rooms, just in case.

Just in case, for example, when one is reading galley proofs of the convention program, a Chicago preacher calls to ask if it will still be possible to schedule a meeting on problems in religion. "We've heard about your convention and thought it would be helpful if we could meet with your group. Maybe 25 or 30 of us would attend." As the idea was a good one, I thumbed the master schedule. "I can get a room for you on Saturday, the last day, at 2:00. It's the only slot we have left."

"We'll take it," he said. "We'll just have to start working earlier on our Sunday sermons."

"Why don't you tell your group to come to the convention earlier? Give us names and addresses and we'll mail copies of the program and, just this once, guest admission tickets."

That program was the origin of "Speech for Religious Workers," which became one of our Interest Groups and eventually a separate organization, The Religious Speech Communication Association, which continued to meet with us.

Nearly always we had to make compromises. At one hotel I told the sales manager we needed one more medium-sized meeting room than he had shown me. He shook his head, but finally said: "Well, there's always the Topaz. It's really a skating rink, but sometimes we use it as a meeting room."

We took a look at it. Basically it was a small, oval, arena, wrapped around on three sides by tiers of seats. Perhaps fifty people could be accommodated. A speaker would have to turn his head from one far side to the other in order to make eye contact with listeners. Slender pillars rooted among the tiers made certain seats even more undesirable. I accepted it, but hoped we would not have to use it extensively. During the convention I looked in on one of the meetings there, and shuddered.

SALES MANAGERS invariably quizzed me about "food functions," their money makers. What breakfasts, luncheons, dinners, could they serve us? What cocktail parties could they schedule?

I flunked an interview with the sales manager of Chicago's elegant Sherman Hotel. "Will you have a convention dinner?" he asked. "No," I said, "a convention luncheon."

"That's bad."

"What's bad about it?"

"We serve luncheons at $3.50 up. But our dinners are $5 up. We would love to serve you a nice convention dinner."

"We can't afford a nice convention dinner. We would like a nice convention luncheon, although a fair number of our people will not eat here but will come in later for the program."

"Where will they eat?"

"Oh, they'll go outside to a modestly priced restaurant, White Castle, or drug store counter."

"That's not too good. Well, will you have a cocktail party?"

"Oh, no, we never have cocktail parties. Many of us will go to the small parties that the publishers have, which are free."

"Will you have smaller groups, like alumni groups, that will have luncheons?"

"Yes, we'll have half a dozen alumni luncheons—University of Michigan, University of Wisconsin, Ohio State University, and others—but out of the hotel, which is cheaper. I'll get a list of nearby restaurants that have a special room and advise them as to menus and prices."

"That's really bad. Let me tell you, professor, we'll have the Scrap Iron Institute of America meet with us and they'll have half a dozen big dinner gatherings that will start at 5:00 and last until midnight. Well, what drinking will you do?"

"I'll have a small party in my room and so will other people. I'll bring a bottle from home. We'll finish by 6:00 so our folks can grab a sandwich nearby and then take in a theater."

He flashed me a now-I've-heard-everything look. In return I gave him my money-is-not-everything speech: "A hotel is a social institution. Its purpose is to serve the public. Often the impression that visitors get of a city is the impression they get of the hotel. Our people come from schools, colleges, universities, clinics, broadcasting studios. Our job is to teach young people. We are ladies and gentlemen. We have class. At the end of the year you should be able to tell your directors that not only scrap iron executives but also teachers have enjoyed the hospitality of the Sherman." I didn't budge him.

I didn't concoct that speech out of thin air. On a previous occasion I had learned that a sales manager was considering two groups that sought the same weekend, and that, although the other was larger, he preferred us. "Why do you say that?" I asked, puzzled. "The other group will bring more people."

"Well, our network of sales managers gets reports on conventions. Staffs of other hotels tell us that your people are fine to have around. If you want this hotel, just say so and I'll write you in."

I remembered his kind words and wondered if they were mere sales talk. Later I picked up a remark that made me feel he had spoken in earnest. A group of speech teachers was in an elevator, and the operator asked: "Who are you folks? What group is it that is meeting in the hotel this week?"

"We're speech teachers," one of the women told him.

"Well, well. I'll have to say this; you are the nicest people we have had since the undertakers' convention."

One year while casing the spanking-new Statler Hotel in Los Angeles, I lingered in the big ballroom where the Dancemasters of America were holding what they had billed as a business session. I saw five hundred attractive and shapely men and women, in shorts or slacks, standing in neat rows, practicing a new dance step called the London cuddle. It all seemed useful and helpful, and although I was not used to this sort of business meeting, I did not want to dismiss a new idea hastily, and filed the notion for future consideration.

Sometimes I looked in on conventions of other groups, to see if their problems were different from ours.

I was in a Chicago hotel and as I walked up and down the halls, I noted a sign in front of the Lake Michigan Ballroom indicating that a convention of what I will call the National Association of Chocolate Candy Manufacturers was in progress. Bridling with curiosity, I went in to see how this group operated.

A man was up front strumming a guitar as members filed in. That struck me as a nice touch and I fantasized starting our general session with a guitar player. "Before we hear our keynote address from President Thomas A. Rousse, here are a few numbers from Chet Atkins . . ."

The first speaker was a representative of the Fanny Farmer company (now I'm guessing) and he told what a problem they had selling chocolates in the summer time. In that age, before air conditioning, their nice chocolates melted before the customer could get them home, making them less attractive.

The next speaker came from the Martha Washington people and she said that the country was going diet crazy and people were buying fewer Martha Washington chocolates because they were fattening.

The third speaker, from Russell Stover's, talked about importing chocolate and how the prices were steadily increasing. After all, they don't grow cocoa beans in Chicago.

I could stand no more of the gloom, and left. It's clear, I mused, that all groups have problems. Speech teachers, at least, don't have this particular set. Whatever it is we do, we do it as well in summer as in winter. Whatever it is we do, it's not fattening. And whatever it is we do, we do it at home. We're not worried about the import market.[1]

Out of years of attending conventions I discovered the Mellowing Effect. The first few hours of any convention are frustrating: members endure aggravating transportation from the airport to the hotel, long lines and delays in getting rooms—and in a newer age, problems arising from computer breakdowns—slowdowns at the badge desk, initial difficulties in locating rest rooms, elevators, and the meeting rooms themselves. Then people meet people, ancient friendships are renewed, experiences swapped; the Mellowing Effect has started to set in. To this day when I attend a convention and see long, slow-moving lines at the hotel registration desk and the explosive displays of annoyance and frustration, I smile inside myself and think, "Well, well, we're going to have another delightful convention. All the signs are in place."

ONE REASON I have enjoyed watching hotels change and improve over the years is that I have seen seven decades of the business of providing lodging. I missed the stagecoach phase and the early part of the train phase, but came in as the automobile was beginning to take over.

I met the first generation of auto tourist facilities in the 1920s, when I was a high school senior at Osceola, Iowa. Many municipalities had erected, in the center of town, a "tourist camp," a cluster of small buildings with a central shelter that contained shower, lavatory, and toilet facilities. Beds and mattresses were provided, but travelers brought their own bedding. No charge was made, the townspeople anticipating that visitors would spend a few dollars with the nearby merchants. These camps were popular, since tourists would not have to pitch a tent on some farmer's pasture and sleep on collapsible army cots.

Imagine scheduling a convention in the 1990s and advertising, "Free lodging nearby. Beds and mattresses provided. Bring your own soap and blankets."

In 1947 I was invited to teach in the summer session at the University of Southern California. We tuned up the eight-year-old Chevy and spent four days, mainly on Old 66, and met the second generation of tourist facilities. Just as drivers had steadily demanded better roads, they had also insisted on convenient parking and beds already made up; they wanted to "come as you are"; they did not want to be bothered with bellboys and tips. Costs were moderate, substantially less than the $2 or $2.50 a night that hotels in towns and cities were charging for a single.

I remember a Mom and Pop place, maybe in New Mexico, maybe in Arizona; at night the states all look alike. We arrived just behind two other cars, and I walked to the front door just behind their drivers. We had been on the road all day; I was too tired to contemplate driving to the next town; I was suddenly, completely drained. Mom, in the doorway holding a fistful of bills, ascertained the needs of those just ahead of me, took their money, and indicated their places for the night. After this rush, I caught her eye and asked: Would she still have room for six bodies, this late? Yes, she smiled, she could take the six, though she would need to scatter us about a bit; for this de luxe attention she thought three dollars for the group would be about right.

Hurrying back to the car, I waved an OK at my weary companion, and we carried in the luggage. While she viewed the rooms and mentally apportioned the bodies, I returned to the car and inspected the back seat. Legs and arms were completely tangled; squabbles over territory had long been settled. I selected a limp torso, sorted out its parts, threw it over my shoulder, carried it inside, dumped it on the indicated bed, and returned for another. Gus stripped off such clothes as necessary, helped half-awake sleepers into nighttime attire, and in minutes lights were out. In the morning we gathered around a little table for corn flakes and such, and recycled ourselves for the new day's journey.

What a long ways from Gold Card facilities. No-wall-to-wall carpet, no telephone, no tumbler wrapped in glassine paper, no basket of fruit or bottle of wine, no turning down of the covers at night with a mint on the pillow, no bar or restaurant or pool on the premises. If I am tolerant of crowds at convention hotels and misplaced reservations it is partly because I grew up in the Mom and Pop age.

Beginning in the 1950s a third set of tourist facilities became popular, calling themselves "motels," "motor inns," or "motor lodges." Hotels and motels began to resemble one another in form and function; hotels provided handy parking, and motels went into the convention business. Both organized into chains, each unit linked to the others by a communication network so that "guests"—no longer called "tourists"— could make reservations nationally and internationally. In these developments America was far ahead of the rest of the world.

In the 1980s we could make confirmed reservations in fancy places—the Washington Hilton, the Denver Sheraton, the New Delhi Intercontinental—or we could select our accommodations along the way—the modest local motel or one linked to a franchise. Or, overseas, we could select the bed and breakfast in the English countryside, in Brussels the well-worn hotel across from the railway station, in Copenhagen a hotel booked last-minute at the tourist center. We could get the native experience and not a facsimile of something back home. Way to go! Avoid the elegant establishments! (Still, I personally like the Imperial in Tokyo [Frank Lloyd Wright], the Grand Hotel in Taipei [a wild dream in gold and red], the Raffles in Singapore [dinner outdoors, lanterns, enchanting Oriental music], the Ephesus in Izmir [pools, fountains, attentive waiters]).

So I never got the Gold Card out of my system, but I would abandon it forever in exchange for an evening with the family at a place marked "Cabins." The hotel-motel business in the '40s and '50s had a flavor all its own.

IN 1947 UTAH OBSERVED the centennial of the year when Brigham Young, at the head of his emigrant train, gazed at the future site of Salt Lake City and said, "This is the place."

Long previously, Lowell Lees, head of the University of Utah's speech and theater department, had extended the Association an invitation to meet in Salt Lake City. To offset the inevitable reduced attendance, the Utah department secured a grant of $1,000 from the state's centennial committee to help us meet expenses. On our part, realizing that a meeting in Salt Lake City would stimulate interest in our discipline in the West, we agreed to come. We had not been west for fifteen years, when a convention in Los Angeles had attracted 400 people. Our 1946 Chicago convention had drawn nearly 1,400.

Those years long-distance winter travel was by train. A University of Washington professor—Horace Rahskopf, for example, or Laura Crowell—would travel two days to Chicago and spend another twenty hours to get to a New York meeting. And even as late as 1947, postwar travel was still clogging the trains. I wondered about the problem of persuading our eastern, midwestern, and southern members to endure the hardships of a day or two-day trip to Salt Lake City, under crowded holiday conditions, and decided that the answer was to organize a special train.

Studying the railroad map, I wrote to Union Pacific officials to see if they would be interested. They probably wouldn't be; already they had all the business they could handle, and our meeting was to be at the time of heavy Christmas travel; still, it wouldn't hurt to inquire. Expecting a "We're terribly sorry, but no" letter from an underling, I was surprised to hear from the chief passenger agent himself, who offered to come to Columbia personally to discuss the plan.

In our Switzler Hall office, I spread a map of the United States between us and explained where our population centers were, and how many passengers we might anticipate. In minutes we were in the midst of an animated conversation; we decided, at this meeting at the summit, to have not one special, but two:

the first to originate in Chicago, to collect eastern and northern members; the second in St. Louis, to attract the south and southeast. Each train would be all-Pullman, with club car and diner; the basic fare would include an upper berth, or, for a slight premium, a lower. For $98, for example, one could take the day-and-a-half ride from Chicago to Salt Lake City in a lower berth. Round trip. For a little less, from St. Louis.

These would be the first all-speech trains in the history of the universe. Officers and council members were urged to board the St. Louis train, so we could have lofty discussions of policy enroute.

On December 26 our Columbia delegation rode the Wabash Cannonball up the spur to Centralia and greeted the St. Louis special, its steam locomotive pulling ten Pullmans. By that time fifty or sixty were already aboard and we had a hilarious reunion. The journey would be even more exciting than we anticipated. In Kansas City we tripled our crowd, and late at night started the long run to Utah. Others boarded along the way. Meanwhile the Chicago special steamed westward by way of Omaha.

I am saddened to report that, instead of the all-steel cars we had been promised, our Pullmans were creaky, wooden coaches. The purple velour of the seats was worn to the nap. Cars weaved and chandeliers swayed. The steam lines supplied too much heat at some times and not enough at others. The water in the drinking fountains tasted rusty. But no one really minded. The war was just barely over, and no one was used to elegance.

That evening and next day we had council and committee meetings on the new constitution, members taking as active a part as officers, and by journey's end we had not only revised the constitution but had also dreamed up other ventures. Surely on that memorable trip brainstorming was invented.

As planned, the two trains arrived at Salt Lake City within minutes of each other; Chicago train on one track, St. Louis train alongside. Three hundred teachers crowded the platform. A swarm of taxis got us to the Hotel Utah; the local committee had been atop every detail. Sunday afternoon we were in the Tabernacle, where we had a reserved section as guests, to hear the *Messiah*. Handel's music is inspiring even if rendered by high school musicians, but as it poured from the vast choir and augmented orchestra, in the acoustically-graced Tabernacle, it was magnificent.

My job as executive secretary now shifted into high gear. Luckily we had put into effect pre-registration procedures which, even this first time, worked well. Those who had not pre-registered and were standing in the longer line, saw the advantage of the plan. Though one of Murphy's laws is that "the other line is moving faster," in this instance it actually was.

Many western members paid their fees in silver dollars. I knew about this custom, having grown up with it in Gilman City, and it sank in when, late each night, I had to pack a bag of heavy silver dollars to my hotel suite. Next day I personally carried them to the Bank of Utah and exchanged them for a cashier's check, an action I was to regret in that future decade when silver prices exploded. I should have kept those lovely silver dollars, no doubt most of them Morgans, and in exchange given the Association a personal check. With the profits from that and a few similar ventures I could have bought my own bank.

President Magdalene Kramer, of Teachers College, Columbia University, presided over a fine program. As the Association had had only three women presidents in its three decades, she felt that the prestige of women everywhere was at stake. Members of the University of Utah speech and theater department—Lees, Halbert Greaves, Wallace Goates—rounded up special attractions. We perfected our new constitution and initiated other enterprises.

At midafternoon of December 31 we looked forward to the departure of the two specials at 6:00. When I realized we would spend New Year's eve on the train, I visited the state liquor store to buy provisions for the celebration. Everybody else, will forget this necessity, I reasoned, so it is up to me to act. An executive secretary is one who thinks of everything; that's what "executive" means.

I had hardly entered the store when in came W. Norwood Brigance, past president. He, too, was far-sighted. Among other items he bought a bottle of White Horse scotch. As we were sacking our purchases, Alan Monroe, also a past president, arrived on a similar thoughtful mission. I hardly need add that these gentlemen were authors, researchers, alert thinkers.

When the two trains pulled out they carried exhilarated but exhausted passengers. On each train we opened windows, easily done on old coaches, and waved back and forth. Gradually the Chicago train angled to the north and we to the south.

AT THE CONVENTION some one had told the hoary story about the president of Northwestern University who had been pressured by the alumni to confer an honorary degree on a horse. This horse, he had been assured, was no ordinary animal; it had, in fact, played third base for the Brooklyn Dodgers. Reluctantly the president agreed, and at the commencement ceremony he concluded the presentation with this observation: "This is the first time, ladies and gentlemen, that I have ever presented an honorary degree to a whole horse."

As we rode homeward, some one suggested that we organize a group, The Ancient and Honorable Order of the Whole Horse—a concept that was received with wild applause.

You can imagine how bright, limber, and fertile minds, like Brigance, Monroe, Kramer, Bower Aly, T. Earle Johnson, Karl Wallace, Giles Wilkeson Gray, Leslie Irene Croger, could take a gimmick like this and run with it, especially when in a mellow state of mind. Those in our Pullman collected under the chandelier, everybody eager to contribute. When Brigance proposed that his bottle of White Horse become our icon, he was greeted with cheers. When Wallace added that each member should write his or her initials on the bottle label, the proposal was approved with a roar. When Gray added that said initials, however, should never deface the image of the horse itself, but be inscribed elsewhere on the label, we respected the wisdom of this honorable parliamentarian. Every idea seemed inspired.

Our black porter, Arnold, started making up berths at the far end of the car, getting closer and closer to our group in the center. We persuaded him to leave unmade the berths around us, for the moment; he agreed, but departed, shaking his head.

We concocted an oath—the oath of Horsetotle, an ancient Greek. We pledged undying loyalty and declared we would be willing to be beat with a crupper if ever we betrayed a secret. We wrote a song—the tune bore a surprising resemblance to that old rouser, "The More We Get Together, the Happier We'll Be." (It continued: "For your stable will be my stable, and my stable will be your stable.") Eventually we printed and distributed membership cards, to be carried on the person at all times. Failure to carry the card subjected the delinquent to a fine of a bushel of oats.

We avoided writing a constitution—we had already had too much of that—-but elected officers. Everybody became not only a Founding Fodder or a Founding Mudder, but also an officer. Aly became Exalted Grand Fodder. Brigance, Chief Horse Thief. I, naturally, Master of De Tails. Kramer, Pride of the Stable. James H. McBurney, Exalted Neigher. E. C. Buehler, Lord Adjuster of the Crupper. Hattie Irene Jones, Reckless Rider of the Range. We created a Committee on Halterations. We devised a ritual on the spot, and administered it to everybody in the car; then we invaded other cars, processing the entire trainload except those who had unwisely gone to bed.

Arnold came by to prepare the rest of the berths but again we waved him off.

Just before midnight we broke open the bottles we had shrewdly purchased and served the beverage in waxed paper cones snitched from the car's drinking fountain. At midnight we sang "Auld Lang Syne" and again, "The More We Get Together." We sang Christmas songs, popular songs we had grown up with, songs of three wars from "Tenting Tonight" to "Over There" to "Don't Sit Under the Apple Tree." Eventually our numbers dissolved and Arnold finally made up the rest of the berths.

Outside a violent blizzard was raging. Snow had drifted over the tracks; the speed of the train had steadily decreased. Our Louisiana, Arkansas, and Alabama friends feared they would miss their connections in Kansas City. When I carried their worries to the conductor, he reminded me that the safety of the train and its passengers was his first responsibility, and that the speed of the engine was determined by the length of clear track that the engineer could see ahead. "We have two men in front of the engine, carrying lanterns; they are walking every foot of the track, and will not let the train proceed until they have inspected the rails." We were hours late getting into Kansas City. Missing connections no longer worried us.

For the next few years the Ancient and Honorable Order held an initiation meeting at the annual convention, late on the second night after the theaters had let out. I always arranged in advance with the sales manager to let us have a room far removed from the sleeping areas, so that our hilarity would not disturb other guests. Invitations to join were freely extended. And we automatically took in spouses, who enjoyed the fun. Anybody could bring a friend, who would be promptly initiated into the Order. Occasionally we roped in such dignitaries as the mayor of the convention city or the president of a hotel chain. They took the oath, signed the bottle, and without too much difficulty learned the song; they received a membership card and were cautioned about the necessity for carrying it at all times.

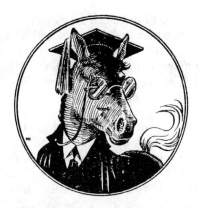

Younger professors heralded their initiation as a turning point in their careers, indicating that they had finally arrived. But I must admit that with few exceptions the new members did not get the same thrill that we had that first night, on that weaving, groaning, yellow, Union Pacific Pullman, when the purple velour was handsome and we felt no pain, despite the blizzard that swept the western plains. And as the founders themselves got older and found it less amusing to stay up late after two full days of conventioning, the ceremonies that once seemed so imaginative lost their sparkle. The Order died almost as quickly as it was born. But as the half-soused fraternity pledge who was arrested for climbing up a sorority fire-escape remarked, it seemed like a good idea at the time.

WHEN MY FIRST TERM of office ended, the campuses were still so crowded, and the possibility of finding another university that would provide office space was so remote, that I had agreed to continue another three years; but after six years I knew I must turn to other projects. Orville Hitchcock of the University of Iowa was elected to take over the national office, beginning in 1951.

On a happy July 1 a vast Allied Van drove to the front door of Switzler Hall and four uniformed men loaded three electric typewriters, four filing cases, the fertile Robotyper, a new addressing machine, a postage meter with envelope-sealing capability, baskets of multicarbon placement forms, 6,000 back issues of journals, records showing that income had nearly tripled, six geese a-laying, ten lords a-leaping, and twelve drummers drumming, and thus the Association could move on to higher levels of vision and prosperity. And in the Artcraft Press basement was the remainder of a carload of book paper, and half a ton of lead slugs, wrapped in page-size chunks—the 1950 *Directory*, ready for the updating process that would turn it into the 1951 *Directory*.

I could settle down to pick up the bolt ends and remnants of my academic career. Instead of a Gold Card bastard I could become a Library Card gentleman. I could resume the study and writing that had been sidetracked by six years of managing business details and directives of a national association.

I did have a lingering regret. When I lost the Association's furniture, fixtures, and responsibilities, I also lost the six talented young women with whom I had worked so long. Weeks before, we had explored the options that would be available to them when the Association left Columbia. Through the University's personnel office we helped them secure positions for the time remaining before their husbands graduated. As I write this I am haunted by names, faces, of those who had helped over the years: Kathryne, Barbara, Thelma, Helen, Connie, Ginny, Amelia, Mary, Dark-Eyes. I do not recall all the last names, but I recall their faces and many things they did. And Bonnie McElhiney, secretary to the Department in its third-floor office, who often helped with a first-floor rush. I can still see stacks of incoming and outgoing mail, proofs, forms, records, folders, bills and invoices, the stream of callers: candidates, deans, department heads, superintendents and principals, the auditor, the man from Union Pacific, the visiting firemen. (You're still wondering about Dark-Eyes? I'm amazed that I've forgotten her name, considering all she did for us. Slender, lovely, quiet, versatile, ready to help, she ran the office's first IBM Executive Electric, the model with variable spacing that made a letter look like print.)

I wish I had taken a staff picture. I wish I had had an occasional Christmas or birthday party. I wish I had installed coffee breaks, which became immensely popular after the war. But I wasn't used to coffee breaks, and neither was the staff. I remember only a single social gesture—from Salt Lake City I brought them an enormous, 15-pound, 15-dollar box of assorted chocolates, from a candy factory recommended by the local people. They loved the chocolates and shared them with the mail man and graduate students and teaching assistants.

Bonnie handled the mail that continued to drift in after the office had moved. Much of it she forwarded routinely, but occasionally she showed me an oddity: for example, the letter from the Chicago magician who offered to saw a lady in half at the 1952 convention. This being an election year, we forwarded it to the new secretary, with the thought that he confer with the magician who had written us about causing an elephant to vanish. Another letter was from Tim's Lobster House of Augusta, Maine, who wrote that his city would be a good locale for our next convention, and that he would like to invite the recipient and his lady to Augusta for a complimentary lobster dinner to discuss the matter.[2]

RESUMING A FULL-TIME professorial career was not a simple on-line process. As soon as the 1951 summer session was over, and with a six-week interval before school resumed, I conferred with Gus and the four kids at Mortgage Lane, the name we always gave to wherever we lived. I suggested I would like to retire to the upstairs study-bedroom, to draft the manuscript that became *Teaching Speech*. If, I said, I could be freed from doing the things that professor-type fathers and husbands usually did in late summer, like painting the house or fixing screens or going on picnics and swims at Stephens Lake, I would work diligently on this manuscript. If, however, they happened to see me sprawled over the bed, as if napping, they were to say to themselves: our loved one is not sleeping; he is meditating about a chapter. As a reward, if all worked well, Next Summer I would be at their complete disposal.

The arrangement was not a bad one; they left me to my own devices, especially in the morning, and I managed to be something of a companion, occasionally in the afternoon. I assembled notes and materials from having taught in high school in Vermillion and Kansas City, from supervising practice teachers and teaching speech education in Syracuse. I wrote to friends to get copies of syllabi, to state associations to get copies of the new courses of study that were appearing, to principals to get information about qualifications, ratings, and salaries. I wrote for beginning teachers because, as I explained in the Foreword, all my life I had been a beginner. By early fall I had written a first draft; for me a first draft is a monumental achievement.

In December I made arrangements with Heath Meriwether to print the manuscript. He worked the job in and around the journals and other stuff he was doing, and the book came out in March. It was fun to prepare ad copy for speech journals, to send out desk and review copies, to prepare circulars for direct mailing. The fourth edition, published by McGraw-Hill, appeared in 1971.

Working with Heath, discussing printing, mailing publicity materials, ogling a budget, made me feel that in a way I had not left the Association-managing business after all. Or put it the other way: in the midst of Association responsibilities I had always been a Speech Teacher.

10

Diamond Crystals

THE SPEECH COMMUNICATION ASSOCIATION celebrated its Diamond Anniversary in San Francisco, November 1989, a few days after the great earthquake. SCA was modest about its birthday: a couple of all-convention parties, a bit of picture taking, a brunch with champagne, the usual reunions of college and university graduates, occasions featuring members who had been present, more or less, since the creation. 1989 was an anniversary to be observed, but it was also a year out of which anniversaries will be born: the year The Wall was breached, the year that Eastern Europe, country by country, declared an end to the Cold War.

Seventy-five is a vaster figure than appears at first glance. In America it is the span of an average lifetime; it is more than a third of the age of the Republic itself. Go back one seventy-five year period and you are in the decade that saw the sinking of the *Titanic*, fought World War I, made the first transcontinental telephone calls, heard the voices of Bryan, Wilson, and Darrow. Go back two seventy-five year periods and you are in the 1830's, listening to Clay, Webster, and Calhoun; eventually they would debate whether a Union of 26 states can hang together. If you want transportation, there's the stage coach and the Erie Canal. If you want communication, you can yell or send smoke signals or write a letter and send it at the speed of a person on foot, on horseback, or on a sailing ship. After a diamond anniversary, we are entitled to a few musings. Reflections. Crystals.

AN ASSOCIATION'S NATIONAL STAFF often thinks about the rank and file, the people who do not hold offices or write articles but pay dues, scan journals, attend meetings, mark ballots. This statement is true whether it applies to the Modern Language Association of America, much older than we (founded 1883), with 27,500 members, or to the American Association of University Professors (1913) with 50,500, or to us (1914) with 6,700.

In the days when a first-class letter could be sent for 4c and bulk mail for less, the Association did much direct mailing in connection with membership drives. We would stuff and sort the envelopes, tie them in bundles, put them in heavy canvas sacks, and lug them to the postoffice. Then we would await the returns. As the envelopes began to come back, Connie or Thelma or Helen or Dark-Eyes would open them and put the checks and money orders in one stack, the subscription blanks or directory entries in another. Often I would riffle through the checks, mainly bearing names of men and women I never knew, might not ever know, and say to myself, Well, now we can meet that bill from Artcraft Press or our next payroll. We could never have had much of an organization if we had had only the dues from the Famous People.

Of course there were nagging worries. Any given year, we would lose old members as well as gain new members. Our faces would light up when we would count, for example, 600 new members. Bye and bye we would become aware that during the same period we had had, for example, 500 dropouts. The term for this situation is "float." We saved the type for the *Directory* from one year to the next, so we would not have to reset entries that were unchanged from the year before. Each entry was represented by 1 to 5 strips of lead. At Artcraft Press when the new *Directory* was being assembled, I have watched the foreman riffle through a galley of these lead strips, keep those that could be used again (the faithful, devoted, continuing members) and cast into the "hellbox," to be remelted and recycled, those whose memberships had expired (the dropouts). I have wondered if Jaxson, Arlo, Instr. in Sp. and Debate, Concordia Seminary, Concordia, OH, A.B. Hamilton '47, M.A. Western Michigan '49, grad. stud. U. of Chicago '50-'52, pub. spk., deb., minor Eng., who failed to renew, heard his 4 slugs as they splattered into the hellbox. Later the foreman would insert the shiny, newly minted strips of those that represented the shiny, newly minted members.

In 1969 the Association made a count of the float, and came up with: 1,200 new members, 1,200 dropouts—a gloomy statistic.[1] At the Diamond Anniversary convention of the American Association of University Professors, I visited with the General Secretary and asked him his thoughts on this subject. "The rank and file are our strength," he said, reverently. "We couldn't exist without them." His office processes 50,500 checks a year, give or take a few hundred. Think what a problem he must have, or the National Education Association (1,700,000 members) must have, with float. One answer is that many people need more than one reminder to pay their dues.

Organizations bless the rank and file. Executive Director James Gaudino and his troops, in the headquarters of the Speech Communication Association at Annandale, Virginia, on that street with the funny name, Backlick Road, should say, following Jimmy Durante's lead, not "Thank you, Mrs. Calabash, wherever you are," but "Thank you, John, Mary, Teresa, Manuel, Sammy, et al, wherever you are."

MINNESOTA football coach Bernie Bierman wrote a feature for (let's say) *Collier's Weekly* about how important the backfield was: the quarterback, the halfbacks, the fullback; the running game, the passing game. Just couldn't win without the backfield. Buried in the article, however, was a sentence: "Now you Gopher linemen know I'm just kidding. We'd be nowhere without you."

I've mentioned the rank and file; now I need to mention those who step forward and do necessary chores. Officers, editors, come and go; one finishes a task, and some one else steps forward. The tasks are never easy. And, as *Speech Monographs* editor Russell Wagner once said: "We work for weeks getting out an issue; finally it goes into the mail; but we never seem to know who reads what or likes what." One can ask, Who cares, really? In *A Man for All Seasons*, Robert Bolt writes about young Rich, who regretted that at the new school, he would be a mere teacher.

"Why not be a teacher?" asked Sir Thomas More. "You'd be a fine teacher. Perhaps a great one."

"And if I was who would know it?"

"You, your pupils, your friends, God—not a bad public, that."[2]

Thinking of the problem of being a leader, wondering why people do it if praise is scarce, I conducted a hushed survey of editors: Robert G. Gunderson, Indiana University, who had the unusual experience of editing journals in two disciplines, *Quarterly Journal of Speech* and *Journal of American History*; Walter R. Fisher, University of Southern California, former editor of *Quarterly Journal of Speech*; and John Daly, University of Texas, former editor of *Communication Education*. How arduous is the task? How rewarding?

Well, we're talking about 500 to 800 manuscripts submitted during a three-year term; an acceptance rate of from 20% to less than 10%; the fact that few articles are printed exactly as submitted, that every article has to be read at least once, and that promising articles are given six or seven readings, by the editor, an associate editor, or others. Certain correspondence is required, including, occasionally, writing a note of rejection to a respected colleague.

I tried to visualize 800 manuscripts—the term-paper output of 80 seminars, each with 10 students. Were there rewards? Here's Gunderson: "Editors get better at their jobs with experience. . . . I became adept at suggesting alternative outlets for many items, thus softening the agony of rejection. . . . There is little praise or blame for editors, but authors often were grateful for editorial improvements." Here's Fisher: "All in all, with all this, I treasure my experience as editor. I hope it was worth while for others as well." Here's Daly: "I was constantly surprised, pleased, amazed, saddened, and even sometimes bewildered by the discoveries I made during my tenure. . . [Yet] the rewards very much outweighed the costs."

I might have surveyed Association presidents, each of whom also serves a three-year term, beginning with being second vice-president. And much of this narrative has described the activities of an executive secretary. In office-holding there is an agony-to-ecstasy ratio, itself a kind of float. At times there is more agony than ecstasy; at other times the opposite. In the short term, agony persists, ecstasy wears off. Alfred Lunt and his wife Lynn Fontaine were a brilliant team on stage and in the cinema. On one occasion, Alfred was heaping Lynn with compliments; then he said, casually, as a brief aside, "In one scene you didn't seem to have any lips"; then another round of even gaudier and more exquisite compliments. Lynn, reflecting a second or so, said: "No lips, eh?" In the long term, however, the complaints fall to the wayside, the glow of professional friendship continues.

Any group needs its leaders and it needs its rank-and-file. It couldn't exist without both.

WHAT MAY BE OVERLOOKED is that leaders and the rank-and-file need the Association. At the outset, state and regional associations received support from the national office, as already mentioned: publicity in journals, discussion in Council meetings, space on convention programs, publication of special projects.

The Association has liaisons with other national organizations and national officers. A single issue of *Spectra* mentioned the Association of School Boards (nation-wide classroom news programming), the Association for Supervision and Curriculum Development (improvement of oral communication instruction), the American Association for the Advancement of Science (of which it is an affiliate) (publication of research papers), members of the U. S. Congress and Senate (the President's national education agenda).[3]

The Association is also on hand for emergencies. Once when high school debate directors got in such serious trouble with North Central, a powerful accrediting agency, that it seemed high school debating might be outlawed, representatives from North Central and the Association worked out a solution in Columbia over a grilled steak supper. When a department gets hauled over the coals (or is in good shape but wants to be better), local people know they can get help from the national office. And how could any teacher, needing a job, or having one but needing an outlet for publishing research, or needing a better job, compete without the help of a professional association?

So it is not always what it can do for us, but what we can do for it. To some students, teachers can talk about teaching in general. To others they can talk specifically about teaching communication, maybe also distributing promotional material from Backlick Road.

I have mentioned previously the steady growth of the Speech Communication Association, despite the fact that a large theater association, a large speech pathology-audiology association, and several smaller associations, have been carved out of it. SCA is not like the American Association of University Professors or Phi Beta Kappa. Our state and regional groups are not "chapters" in a national structure. Each one is fiercely independent; it grew up that way. Many associations interested in communication, state, regional, and national, compete with us for the same people. One ponders whether these could be reunited under a common umbrella, to the good of all.

Perhaps more people should write about the operation of learned societies. In the midst of a book about the nature of science, its limits and its whence and whether, the author, co-recipient of a Nobel prize, discusses Great Britain's Royal Society, which already has observed four centennials and headed for its fifth. What is the usefulness of societies? asks the author. And how can they perpetuate themselves? keep from being too large or too small? honor people in the prime of their careers? avoid overlooking deserving people?[4]

What the leaders and the rank-and-file do for the profession is not something to be done only once, at the start of the school year in August 1991, for example. Immediately in the future are August 1992, August 1993, August 19xx . . . August, August, August. New students, who know not Joseph, will appear on tomorrow's August.

MAINLY, HOWEVER, the question is not alone who does what for whom, but what happens when we meet together. I have discussed conventions before but I cannot entirely shake the topic out of my head.

We were at a conversational bridge party where the players interrupt the playing to exchange a recipe or to comment on Saturday's game. My friend in mathematics slowed up his card-riffling to say that he had just returned from a convention in San Antonio.

My ears twitched. I had to ask: "What did you do there?
"I read a paper."
"How did it go?"
"Fine, I guess. People said they liked it."
"How'd you like San Antonio?"
"Terrible place. Terrible convention. Buzzed in, read my paper, and buzzed out." He snapped the cards in a final, definitive shuffle.

My mind left the bridge table to reflect on the 1979 convention of the Speech Communication Association, in San Antonio. For the first time, there was no headquarters hotel; Executive Director William Work gave us a choice of places to stay, at varying prices. The meetings were well attended and the talk was good; they were held at the new Convention Center, in rooms so compactly arranged that little time was lost in aimless wandering. The walk from the Center to your hotel was probably along the San Antonio River, one of the nation's beautiful strollways. Even late at night, you felt safe and comfortable. If you did not care to walk, you could take a water taxi. You could expose yourself to the Spanish flavor of one of the country's unusual cities. . . . Suddenly my reverie was broken; I heard a faraway voice: "It's your bid . . ."

What, anyway, are the reasons for attending a convention, other than reading a paper? Or seeing the sights? Here is a list:

1. We hear new ideas before they appear in print; ideas that are new to us, even though they have been known for a time to specialists in other areas of our discipline.

2. We discover new books, and teaching materials such as computer programs, which give us ideas for research and for classroom assignments.

3. We renew acquaintances with former friends and make new ones. We meet well-known members of the profession.

4. Small schools often do not have enough teachers in any one area to spark each other. At a meeting we can climb out of our ruts, shatter our established routines, reappraise our personal goals, open new doors that will never be closed.

5. We undergo an intellectual dialysis that dislodges hardened concepts and renews our vitality. We come back with energy we didn't know we had. We catch fire from the enthusiasm of others.

I will omit the disappointments, the dull moments—they abound in all sorts of conventions in all sorts of business and professional fields. Not every paper rings the bell. If you have gone to two conventions, and your friend has gone to twenty, he or she has heard ten times as many bad presentations as you have heard. But here's a menu, somewhat edited, from the viewpoint of this convention watcher: a good paper here and there, a glimpse now and then of a bright and fertile mind, the moving experience of "discovering" a promising newcomer, a stroll through the exhibits to finger the texts, a hundred now for every score that used to be, and once that dinner in a family-style Greek restaurant with half a dozen friends responding to a piano player and one-time popular tunes that finally swept the diners in the room into a great circle to sing the melodies through their smiles and tears, and there was the nice lady, a stranger, a total stranger, and her friends, and it seemed as if our group were singing and nodding to her group, reliving young lives that might have identically grown up though a continent apart.

AND YOU MIGHT MAKE—I hate to use the ugly word—"contacts." Some one may contact you about a new job or a new project. Or mention you to a third party, who will contact you. After I had attended twenty conventions, and had become a Full Professor and Department Head, a real sachem, I was contacted by a department head from an eastern university.

He contacted me in the Hotel Pennsylvania lobby. "Hello," he said. "I've been wanting to contact you. I've been following your career."

"That's nice," I said, offering him my warmest handshake.

"We'd like to have you come to our campus for an interview. We have a good team and would like to add you to it. We're on the move. We're getting heavy command support. We're doing exciting things."

"Hm-m, hm-m," I ventured, encouragingly.

"Now what we have in mind is an assistant professorship . . ."

I heard him out, thanked him, promised to talk to my wife, thanked him again, and let the conversation shift to other subjects.

AS A DISCIPLINE, we do have our problems.

My dentist was drilling away on a bicuspid; I could feel him getting close to a sensitive spot. He stopped to say:

"At Rotary yesterday I was talking to an undertaker. He said, 'I do get a little weary at times of working on dead people.'"

"What did you say to that?"

"I told him, I'd like to work on a dead person once in a while. It would be so much easier to work on a dead person than a live one. You need to be so cautious and careful around the live ones. . . . Now I'm going to have one more little go at you and then we'll be through." I prized the fact that he was trained to be very, very careful, especially the next few seconds, especially since he was approaching a sensitive spot, especially on this particular live one.

Everybody has problems, whether they involve live people or dead people. A large midwestern university combined its departments of geography with geology, to the disadvantage, my friend in geography felt, of geography. "They don't understand us," he said. We, too, have lost a few fine departments. Others, however, have stepped in to fill their places.

For decades I have visited with speech department heads, asking the same questions repeatedly: (1) How's enrollment? (2) How's your staff getting along? (3) Are your new Ph.D.'s getting jobs?

Invariably the answers are: (1) increasing, (2) best staff we've ever had, (3) yes, and to good schools. Sometimes I wonder if speech department heads are wholly to be depended upon for precise and impartial judgments, but when I probe with specific questions, I get specific answers.

Here are real, genuine, checkpoint Charlie problems; you can lay them aside those of your own department:

1. Are enrollments increasing? Is there satisfying demand for advanced courses?
2. Can you place your graduates?
3. Can you attract good teachers and hold them?

I take these questions from articles appearing in educational journals. Discipline X, for example, can get enrollments in the beginning course, but there the interest stops. Discipline Y seems to have run its race, to have passed the peak of its popularity. Discipline Z would like more graduate students but has difficulty placing those it has. These do not sound like problems that annoy us, at least not in wholesale fashion.

I'll end in a lighter vein—notes from a student teacher of French:

1st day: Students not doing well in class. Seem to be weak in vocabulary. Informed them that there will be a test over vocabulary tomorrow.

2nd day: Students did not do well on test. Stressed importance of vocabulary. Must make test easier next time.

3rd day: Students did not do well on vocabulary drill. Told them there would be vocabulary test tomorrow. Stressed importance of study.

4th day: Students did poorly on vocabulary test. Worked on vocabulary during class. Assigned another test.

5th day: Made test easier. Students did better.[5]

SPEECH IS an ancient discipline. The *trivium*, grammar, logic, and rhetoric, was the basic division of the seven liberal arts in medieval schools. Going back further, Socrates, Aristotle, and Plato made extensive contributions to the field of speech. Going back still further to the peoples of Asia or Africa, one reads about ancient papyri contain fragments of advice about speaking and listening.

Along the way were great practitioners, such as Demosthenes and Cicero. Later came medieval writers about rhetoric, Longinus and Augustine. The eighteenth and nineteenth century brought the trivium of Blair, Campbell, and Whately, whose books were used as texts in nineteenth century American universities.

At the turn of the century we had a group of teachers, whom I have called, somewhat arbitrarily, the "first generation," who turned from "elocution" as a name for our discipline to "speech." Their students, the second generation, thought of themselves almost from the beginning as "speech" teachers.

Many "speech" teachers wrote books and articles about (a) outstanding speakers or (b) outstanding rhetoricians and rhetorical movements. Thus we thought of Donald Bryant in connection with Edmund Burke; Russell Wagner in connection with Thomas Wilson; Karl Wallace in connection with Francis Bacon; Waldo W. Braden in connection with Southern speakers and issues; Wilbur S. Howell in connection with early British rhetoric. Ralph G. Nichols brought the field of listening to our attention. Elwood Murray brought interpersonal communication to general awareness. We wrote dissertations about Henry Clay or Clarence Darrow or William Jennings Bryan, and when we ran out of people who were nationally known, we turned to speakers with a regional reputation. Pretty rigorously we kept to the point of view that we were writing about these people as *speakers*.

"Speech" teachers also applied what they had learned to current practices and situations. Their students, "speech communication" teachers and "communication" teachers, facing a steadily increasing complexity of society and the influence of the electronic age, reach for still newer kinds of communication problems. Michael Osborn of Memphis State University, in an article in *The Chronicle of Higher Education*, mentions some of these, including, for example, those that inquire into reasons why television is so important in seeking political office.[6] In 1989-1990 observers in ours and other disciplines commented that the revolutions in Europe and Asia and the changes in government that followed were a result of the widespread availability of electronic communication. Then, as new governments struggled with their inherited problems, many saw that good communication, good dialog, was as important as ever. Still others noted that communication about freedom and democracy among people who had not grown up with freedom and democracy was more difficult than most people had realized. No one should be amazed that teachers who have studied the problem of getting messages from an origin to a destination, using words or signs or symbols or objects or vocal tones or bodily movement, adapting and adjusting as necessary, to one another and to the occasion and to the situation, should peer into the newer kinds of communication situations that came along.

My generation of teachers has spent a good part of their lives in the pursuit of eloquence. We have marveled at the brilliance of speakers like Fox, Gladstone, Churchill, Lincoln, Roosevelt, King. And we have been moved by a well-researched seminar report, a plea to a city council, a cogent explanation of the budget by the church treasurer, a talk at the local foreign affairs club, a clear diagnosis by a physician to a worried patient or by a mechanic to a harried driver. All of these are forms of eloquence, a word the root of which is "to speak out."

Research in speech/communication will continue along many lines. And this situation suggests another kind of float: as we increase our interest in some topics, we lose interest in others. We have also noted that if we abandon a field, some one else may move in on it.

WE MADE IT all the way to a Diamond Anniversary, in MCMLXXXIX. We can look ahead to the Millennium, which is MMI, and to the Centennial, which is MMXIV. We travel through the years and decades one I at a time. Hundreds of teachers now in our discipline will be around to see these marvels. Members of other organizations are also thinking these thoughts. The learned societies must be doing some things right.

References and Acknowledgments

References

I consulted *The Past Is Prologue: A Brief History*, edited and written by Robert C. Jeffrey and William Work for the Speech Communication Association's Diamond Anniversary year, for information about publications and special projects. I also consulted older issues of the Association's *Annual Directory* for biographical information and other details.

Some material comes from an unpublished manuscript, *Roving Professor: The Wartime Decades, 1933-1953*, a sequel to the author's *Finally It's Friday*.

Chapter 1: In the Beginning

[1]Basic sources for the National Association of Academic Teachers of Public Speaking are: *English Journal, 3* (1914), 586-589, *4* (1915), 339; *6* (1917), 627; *Quarterly Journal of Public Speaking, 2* (1916), 83-87; *Quarterly Journal of Speech Education, 4* (1918), 235-238. James M. O'Neill's article, The national association, *Quarterly Journal of Public Speaking, 1* (1915), 51-58, is invaluable. Andrew T. Weaver, contemporary of the founders, wrote about them in "Seventeen Who Made History—The Founders of the Association," *Quarterly Journal of Speech, 45* (1959), 195-199. (The O'Neill and Weaver articles are reprinted in *The Past is Prologue: A Brief History*.)

Southern Speech Communication Journal, 47 (1982), 107-134, has articles on O'Neill by James H. McBath; on Winans by Loren Reid; on Wichelns by Carroll C. Arnold; on Baird by Owen Peterson; and an introductory essay by Waldo W. Braden.

Part of the material in this chapter is from a talk given at the Golden Anniversary of the Speech and Theatre Association of Missouri, published in *Missouri Speech Journal* (1983), and from "Convention Magic," *Communication Education 35* (1986), 307-311.

[2]Cumnock: *QJS, 15* (1929), 157.

Quotations from *Hurry Home Wednesday: Growing Up in a Small Missouri Town, 1905-1921*, copyright (c) 1978 by University of Missouri Press, and from *Finally It's Friday: School and Work in Mid-America, 1921-1933*, copyright (c) 1981 by University of Missouri Press, are used by permission of the Press.

[3]Coaching the contestants: *Hurry Home Wednesday*, 176-177.

[4]Debate with Martinsville: *Hurry Home Wednesday*, 179-181.

[5]Enrolling at the University of Iowa: *Finally It's Friday*, 213-214.

[6]Planning to get married: *Finally It's Friday*, 237.

[7]Commencement: adapted from *Finally It's Friday*, 281.

Chapter 2: Rossum's Universal Robots

[1]The word "robot" has an interesting etymology (one ancestor is *arabeit*, trouble, from Old High German). The Czech origin is *robota*, compulsory labor, drudgery.

I dedicate this chapter to high school teachers, who continue the tradition of being not so much specialists but generalists in the field, humanists-without-portfolio.

Chapter 3: Elocution, Speech, Shakespeare

[1]The 1985 government survey referred to is Judi Carpenter's *Trends in Bachelors and Higher Education Degrees, 1975-1985, 12*, published (1987) by the Office of Educational Research and Improvement, U. S. Department of Education. "Communications . . . rose from 18,200 [bachelor's] degrees in 1975 to 40,400

in 1985, a 122 percent increase." The term includes journalism, public relations, etc. as well as general communication, but does not include "communications technology," such as television, radio, and film production, often taught by teachers in our discipline. A better classification would be helpful. See also "A Renewed Teaching Emphasis" by James W. Chesebro in *Spectra*, *25* (1989), 2-3, for other data. Chesebro notes: "A national emphasis on teaching may ultimately reinforce the discipline of communication."

In the ten-year period 1975-1985, bachelor's degrees in communications conferred upon men increased by approximately 50 percent; upon women by more than 300 percent (Carpenter, 40-41).

[2]Henry M. Belden, Fairchild's predecessor as head of the Department of English, was sympathetic to the problems of the four speech teachers in the department. His specialty in literature was the ballad.

[3]Robert L. Ramsay's lexicon of Mark Twain's writing and his dictionary of Missouri place names are widely known. He was a man of wide-ranging interests. For more information about Professors Belden, Ramsay, Fairchild, Weatherly, and others, see Leon H. Dickinson, *An Historical Sketch of the Department of English* (University of Missouri-Columbia, 1986).

[4]At Syracuse University in 1941, I planned a conference and invited O'Neill. Gus said, "Why don't we ask him to bring his wife, and stay with us?" As we had just moved, and the living room was still cluttered with crates and boxes, I asked, "What about all this stuff?" She said: "If the O'Neills have reared six children, they won't even notice a few boxes." Edith O'Neill was completely charming; both were fine conversationalists. At dinner O'Neill told us about the founding of the Wisconsin speech clinic; I have never seen the story anywhere else. After retirement, he lectured to Knights of Columbus groups; when he came to Columbia, I persuaded him to tell our students and faculty about the early days of the national association.

Chapter 4: If You Love 'Em, Join 'Em
[1]The founding of the Central States Speech Association is narrated in *Fanfare for Fifty*, published by CSSA at the time of its Golden Anniversary in 1981. *QJS*, *24* (1938), 707 contains the program of the 1937 convention in Columbia.

[2]The note about Irving J. Lee is based on a memorial by Ernest J. Wrage, *QJS*, *41* (1955), 333-334.

[3]*The Lives of a Cell (New York, Bantom Books, Inc., 1974), 73. And see The Medusa and the Snail* (New York, The Viking Press, 1979): "We [people] are the newest, the youngest, and the brightest thing around," 12-18; "All we have to go by is how we walk, sound, write letters, turn our heads," 115.

Chapter 5: Growth of a Discipline
I scanned the "Forum" and "News and Notes" sections of *The Quarterly Journal of Public Speaking* (later *Q.J. of Speech Education*) (still later *Q.J. of Speech*) for the first 40 years of publication.

A "News and Notes" section for *QJS* first appeared in 1923 and was edited by Lousene G. Rousseau. As editor of this section and later as Speech Editor for Harper she often was a hostess at convention cocktail parties for Harper authors and friends. She was genuinely interested in recording happenings in all aspects of the discipline. Her successors continued the tradition, making "News and Notes" a historical record with an informal, self-disclosure quality: notes about newly established Departments of Speech, new buildings, new theaters or radio studios, newly approved graduate programs, announcements of new state and regional associations (and later of their convention programs, often printed in full). Occasionally a death would be reported (there were not many of us, and most of us were young). Names of those on leave of absence. Names of those who were studying towards, or had received Ph.D.'s, especially if they were well known. Personal items, such as: "James M. O'Neill is not teaching this summer, but is spending the summer in New England with his family, and writing a new text."

I edited news and notes in a different format, "Shop Talk," for *QJS* 1954-1956, during the editorship of Wilbur S. (Sam) Howell of Princeton University. The "Shop Talk" format was used for nine years.

[1]Dates in this section come from a *Journal* issue of that year (or of the preceding year, since the item may be published months after the actual event). One interested in a particular association, or department, will likely find in "News and Notes" not only the year of its founding, but also reports of its later activities.

See also Ronald J. Matlon, ed. *Index to Journals in Communication Studies Through 1985*, published by SCA, for articles about state and regional associations.

During the next decade, many regional and state associations (and Departments of Speech/Communication) will celebrate Golden or Diamond Anniversaries).

[2]Ads for departments\schools of speech or oratory come from the *Quarterly Journal of Speech Education*, as indicated.

[3]More about doctorates: By 1934 (i.e. the first 20 years of the Association's history) Wisconsin had awarded 15; Iowa 14; Cornell 8; Columbia University—Teachers College 5; Michigan 3; Stanford 1. Denver, Illinois, Louisiana, Marquette, Minnesota, Northwestern, Southern California, Syracuse, and Utah reported having given master's degrees during that 1902-1934 period; many from this list would soon be offering the doctorate as well.

By 1954, these schools had also reported awarding doctor's degrees: Colorado State College of Education, Florida, Florida State, Houston, Indiana, Michigan State, Missouri, New York University, Ohio State, Pennsylvania State, Pittsburgh, Purdue, Texas, Washington University, Western Reserve, Yale.

In 1954 a student seeking a doctorate in speech had 30 institutions from which to choose. In 1989, the Diamond Anniversary year, 80 or more.

How many doctorates in speech-theater-speech pathology/audiology have been granted? Knower counted 4,309 through 1968 (*Speech Monographs, 36*). SCA's *Directory of Graduate Programs, 1986-1987*, Table I, vi, shows 3,246, 1969-1985, through 79 departments (pp. 313-315). Total doctorates, 1922-1985, 7,555.

[4]*The Past Is Prologue: A Brief History* is the source of data such as those in this section.

[5]Wiltse statement: *QJS, 26* (1940), xix.

Chapter 6: Teaching Speech: Wartime

[1]*Time*, special issue, Communication 1940-1989, 10-11. Prepared with the assistance of a committee of Speech Communication Association members for distribution at the Diamond Anniversary convention.

[2]Brigance on book review editors: *QJS, 28* (1942), 359-360.

[3]Part of this talk eventually landed in *Finally It's Friday*: writing a newspaper story on a speech without hearing it, 20-22; correcting a Congressional speech after delivering it, before it is printed in the *Record*, 155-156.

[4]Brigance volumes: *QJS, 42* (1956), 104. Hochmuth volume: *idem*, 185.

[5]*History of American Education* was published in 1954 by Appleton-Century-Crofts, Inc. See *The Past is Prologue*, 46, for other publications sponsored by SCA or by subgroups.

[6]Notes on New York State Speech Association: *QJS, 29* (1943), 390; *QJS, 30* (1944), 377-378.

[7]Tolley's efforts to bring Air Force cadets to Syracuse University: *At the Fountain of Youth: Memories of a College President*, Syracuse University, 1989, 77-79.

[8]One result of moving from Missouri to New York was that because of gas rationing and crowded trains we could visit less frequently with our parents in Iowa. We therefore wrote more letters, and from this correspondence I gleaned details about teaching Air Force cadets.

Chapter 7: Teaching Speech: Postwar

[1]Data about the GI Bill of Rights come from: Sidney A. Burrell, "The GI Bill and the Great American Transformation, 1945-1967," *Graduate Journal of Boston University, 15*, 3-10; *Encyclopedia of Education, 4, 134-138; Keith W. Olson, The GI Bill, the Veterans, and the Colleges* (Lexington 1974) (Olson quotes studies indicating the superior achievement of veteran students).

Chapter 8: The Original Gold Card Era

[1]The note about the *Directory* comes from *QJS, 42* (1956), 335-336.

[2]For a note on *The Speech Teacher*, see *QJS, 40* (1954), 99; Waldo W. Braden, The founding of the *Speech Teacher*, *The Speech Teacher, 18* (1969), 151-153 (in this issue are also articles on the founding of *QJS* and *Speech Monographs*).

Chapter 9: Convention Hotels and Other Perils

[1]National Association of Chocolate Candy Manufacturers: Convention magic, *Communication Education*, *35* (1986), 311.

[2]Sawing a lady in half, complimentary lobster dinner: *Quarterly Journal of Speech*, 1954, 233.

A hotel yarn: My first-ever hotel was in Kansas City, with Father and brother Don. The year was 1920; I was 15, Don was 12. Father had proposed that we would leave Gilman City Thursday morning, after the *Guide* was published, and have a long week end in the big city.

We stayed at The Morgan, a three-story hotel on West 9th Street. Father could have secured a room on the top floor for 50c, but he decided it would be wiser to stay on the second floor for 75c. We climbed the stairs and viewed the room: a large bed for the three of us, a chair, a washstand with bowl and pitcher. In a corner of the room next to the window was a coil of heavy rope, knotted every two feet.

Father inspected the rope, uncoiling it and explaining that in case of fire we would throw the free end of the rope out of the window and climb down it. He made sure the other end was securely fastened to the wall, giving the rope a strong tug and inviting us also to give it a try. We had no doubt that in the event of trouble we could make it to the street.

What's to be the guiding rule, conventioner, when you enter your hotel room? Check out the rope.

Chapter 10: Diamond Crystals

[1]Robert N. Hall reported this 1969 figure in *Spectra*, *10* (1974), 2.

[2]*A Man For All Seasons* played in London (that summer Robert Bolt had three plays booked simultaneously). Of these fine performances, the bit that has persisted in my memory is the brief dialog between Rich and Sir Thomas.

[3]*Spectra*, *26*, 6 (1990) 1, 2.

[4]Peter Medawar, *The Limits of Science* (Oxford 1984), 37-39.

[5]French teacher's vocabulary test: *Quarterly Journal of Speech*, *40* (1954), 241.

[6]Osborn, "The Study of Communication Flourishes in a Democratic Environment," *The Chronicle of Higher Education*, *36* (1990), B2-B3.

Acknowledgments

J. Jeffery Auer of Indiana University, Paul H. Boase of Ohio University, and John F. Wilson of Herbert H. Lehman College, CUNY, members of the Speech Communication Association's Diamond Anniversary Committee, read an early draft of this manuscript, offered suggestions, and gave it their approval.

Publication of the completed manuscript was authorized by the Speech Communication Association through its Administrative Committee: Gustav W. Friedrich, president, University of Oklahoma; Mark L. Knapp, first vice president, University of Texas; Dennis S. Gouran, second vice president, Penn State University; Michael M. Osborn, immediate past president, Memphis State University; James L. Gaudino, executive director, National Office; and the following from SCA boards: Pam Cooper, chairperson Educational Policies Board, Northwestern University; John Daly, chairperson Publications Board, University of Texas; Robert K. Avery, chairperson Research Board, University of Utah; Caroline D. Ecroyd, chairperson Finance Board, Temple University; David Zarefsky, member Finance Board, Northwestern University; Carolyn Calloway-Thomas, member Finance Board, Indiana University.

I have consulted with Gaudino, James W. Chesebro, director of education services, and Penny Demo, publications manager, National Office, frequently, and am grateful for photos and other materials provided. Waldo W. Braden, Executive Secretary of the Association 1954-1957, at that time at Louisiana State University, now retired and living in Columbia, has given me more counsel and information than he realizes. Laura Crowell, University of Washington, Robert G. Gunderson, Indiana University, Walter R. Fisher, University of Southern California, John Daly, University of Texas, have helped unpuzzle puzzling matters and have supplied needed information.

About the Author

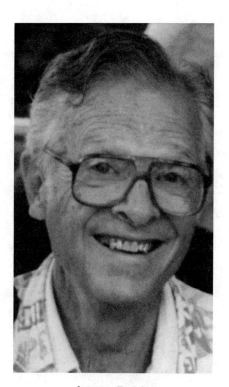

Loren Reid

Loren Reid was Executive Secretary in 1945-1951 of what is now the Speech Communication Association, and was President in 1957.

Reid was awarded the Winans-Wichelns Memorial Award for Distinguished Scholarship in 1969 and the SCA Golden Anniversary Book Award in 1970. In 1981 he received the SCA Distinguished Service Award.

He was a founder of the Speech and Theatre Association of Missouri and founder and first President of the New York State Speech Communication Association and has received distinguished service awards from both associations. In 1937-1939 he was Executive Secretary of the Central States Speech Association. He is a Fellow of the Royal Historical Society.

Reid, Professor Emeritus of Communication at the University of Missouri-Columbia, has received awards from that institution and from Grinnell College for distinguished teaching and service.

Reid's other books include *Hurry Home Wednesday: Growing Up in a Small Missouri Town, 1905-1921* (University of Missouri Press), *Finally It's Friday: School and Work In Mid-America, 1921-1933* (University of Missouri Press), *Speaking Well* (McGraw-Hill Book Company), and *Charles James Fox* (Longmans Green, University of Missouri Press).

Index